Kate!
Be your...
And take goo...
of yoursel...
Robin W Hen...

Women

it's your Turn

By Dr. Robin Hartley

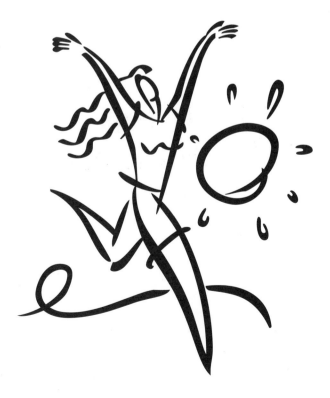

Dedicated to

My family: Bruce, Jonathan, and Christopher
And to my parents: Richard and Shirley

Acknowledgments

The first words written for this book were, "You are great, you can do it!" For weeks the piece of paper containing those words sat on my dining room table waiting for further inspiration. One day, my ten-year-old son noticed that the words were not magically transforming themselves into a book, and said, "Mom, is that it? Are you done? Is that your entire book?" Heartfelt thanks to my husband and two sons for inspiring and motivating me so my dream of writing a women's health book could become a reality.

I wish to thank my father and mother for their support, advice, and the computer skills that they provided.

Thank you to my perimenopausal and menopausal friends and patients who asked for a complete reference guide for their health; they wanted a book that is understandable, easy-to-read, and a quick guide in which they can find answers to the questions that they have about their health and well-being.

I thank Jenny Harle for her good attitude, tireless enthusiasm, and countless hours of typing and retyping the manuscript. Thank you to Julie Ware for her typing of the first chapters. Thanks to Ann Hanigan for her preliminary editing help, and her great sense of humor.

Thanks to Lynn, Tawny, Leigh, Tammy, Olive, Anne, Sandy, Connie, Liz, Melba, and Kris who help define, with grace, a more youthful, healthy, energetic, and vibrant changing face of beauty. Thanks to Amy Acheson, Cosmetologist and licensed Makeup Artist, for the makeup and skin tips.

Thank you to my medical school and residency educators who helped me to understand and appreciate the miracle of the human body.

Thank you to James Patten, M.D., for giving advice on pap smears.

Thanks to Tom and Jodi and Steve and Ann for their expertise and words of encouragement.

Thanks to Denise Sundvold, McMillen Publishing, my editor Bridget, Innova Ideas and Services, and Sigler Printing for their belief in my vision. Thanks to photographer Dave Popelka who took the cover photo and some of the book's interior photos; thanks to Waveland Golf Course for allowing us to hold our photo shoot there.

Thank you Susan Johnson, M.D., for taking time out of your busy schedule to give medical advice on so many key women's health issues—your advice is invaluable, and this book wouldn't have been the same without it.

Introduction
It's Your Turn; Now is Your Time

More than likely, you have held the pause button on your own health and well-being for many years; in that time, you have set your own personal needs aside as you tried to be a good wife, mother, daughter, friend, sister, student, and/or employee.

When you look into the mirror, who do you see? Is the reflection that you see what you had hoped it would be by this time in your life? Have you fulfilled your dreams, accomplished your goals, or created the legacy that you had thought you would have by now?

You will never be as young as you are right now, at this moment. This is your opportunity to take time to reassess where you are in your life and where you want to be 30 years from now. Your future is limited only by your imagination.

This is your chance for a fresh start to being a new and improved you. It is your time to rediscover, reinvent, and reconnect with who you are and what you want to do with your life. Set yourself free from the self-imposed limitations and mental restraints that you have placed on yourself. Learn to scuba dive, go back to school and get a degree, or open your own store. If you can see it and believe in it—then you can achieve it!

In order to be able to enjoy your robust and fabulous future, you will need to have a healthy body. You will want to start to make healthy choices so you will feel and look good from the inside to the outside. To achieve this, you will need your own custom-fit health plan that focuses on prevention and health maintenance.

Congratulations on selecting this book as your women's health guide. This book will provide you with an understandable and easy-to-read reference that will provide answers to the questions that you have about your health; it will provide you with suggestions on how to create a health plan that will give you the steps to better health and a sense of well-being. Learn how to strengthen your body, enrich your mind, and energize your spirit. By balancing your spirit, mind, and body, you can add years to your life, and quality to your years. Enjoy reading your women's health guide. Personalize it to your life.

Celebrate your new beginning and be the best that you can be.

Dr. Robin Hartley

Table of Contents

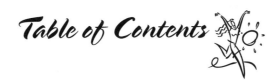

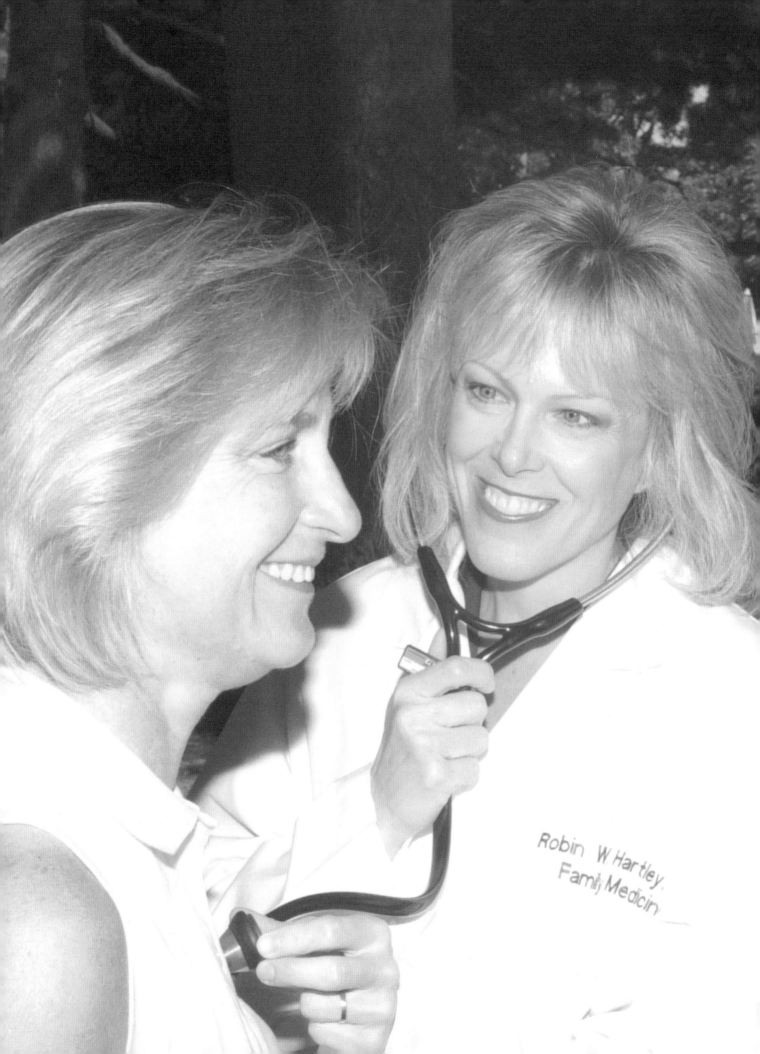

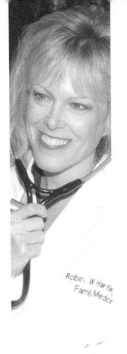

Robin W. Hartle
Family Medicine

Preventive Health Maintenance

YOUR GIFT TO YOURSELF AND YOUR FAMILY

A lot of diseases (your body is at "dis-ease" with itself when you are ill) are preventable and/or treatable when you take charge of your health and well-being. Your goal should be to take simple daily steps to ensure that you are able to live a full, rich, and invigorating life your whole life.

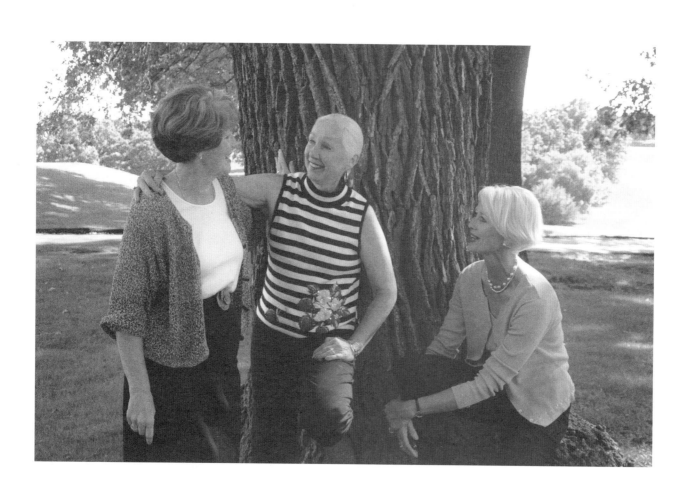

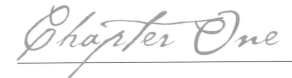

Chapter One

Taking care of your body—if not for you then for those around you—is one of the most selfless and giving things you can do for yourself and your loved ones.

Chapter 1: Preventive Health Maintenance
Your Gift to Yourself and Your Family

Let's face it, you have been on auto pilot for many years when it comes to your own personal health. You skipped your way through your teens and young womanhood with hardly a thought to your health—other than not wanting your period on your honeymoon or wondering whether you or one of your friends would be the first to get pregnant.

While you were trying to get pregnant, and through your pregnancy, you did everything right to ensure a healthy baby. While you were pregnant you quit smoking, decreased caffeine, exercised, and took multivitamins in an attempt to take good care of yourself for your baby's sake.

Or, conversely, you may have plunged head first into your career and kept your tireless energy fueled with the robustness of your social life. You may have even attempted to have it all by juggling babies and a career. Nothing could get in your way or slow you down.

The late (and often sleepless) nights, long work hours, nutrition on the run, and sports activities kept you busy. For most of the time, your body kept up with your frantic pace as you aggressively jumped to the next rung on the ladder of success. You hardly had to give a second thought to your body's upkeep—let alone any preventive health maintenance.

Now is the time for you to start enjoying some of the rewards of a job well done in your life. You have worked hard to get where you are today. You have arrived. In your late 40s and 50s, all cylinders in your life are firing; you are fully energized, empowered, and feeling good. Whatever life has in store for you, bring it on! You are ready for anything. You now have a broader perspective, richer wisdom, a growing family, improved financial position, and a stronger sense of who you are, where you are going, and where you want to be when you retire.

Congratulations on reaching this point in your life. Now is your window of opportunity. You can realign your goals and dreams and make a plan of action with a specific time frame to get you to a healthier stage in your life. Now is your chance. Now is your moment for a fresh start to be who you want to be. This is your opportunity to shower away any self-doubts, self-made limitations, and undermining defeatist attitude that you may have.

Now is also the time when you need to stop for your 100,000 mile health maintenance road check. **Now, more than any other time in your life, you need to stop and look at your lifestyle, risk factors, and family history, and make adjustments to ensure you feel as strong and empowered today as you will be 30 years from now when you are enjoying retirement.** Taking care of your spirit, mind, and body is the most important thing you can do for yourself to ensure a healthy and strong future. Living a preventive and healthy lifestyle, as well as doing daily body maintenance and yearly physicals, is the most selfless thing you can do to ensure your loved ones that you are going to be there for them for the long haul.

What good does it do for you to try to be the healthiest you have ever been while you are pregnant and until your kids are old enough to take care of themselves, if you won't be around long enough for your children's children to know what a wonderful grandmother you will be? Or, what is the point of spending your time choosing a partner and spending years nurturing that relationship, only to be gone before you can enjoy the golden years together? **And why spend years working, saving, and slaving away to have a 401K retirement plan, pension, and investments to secure your financial future if you are not going to be around to enjoy them?**

It could be thought of as selfish to go full throttle now, running through your life with your tires threadbare and your wheels ready to fall off, and not do a few small road checks along the way to ensure your body's high performance in the future. **Right now is the time to take a few moments each day to maintain this magnificent gift of life and this wonderful body you have been blessed with. Taking care of your body, if not for you then for those around you, is one of the best things you can do for yourself and your loved ones.**

A lot of diseases (your body is at "dis-ease" with itself when you are ill) are preventable and/or treatable when you take charge of your health and well-being. Your goal should be to take simple, daily steps to ensure that you are able to live a full, rich, and invigorating life. It is especially important to find a doctor you can call your own and, together, form a partnership.

Now is the time in your life that you need to look at your family history, lifestyle, and modifiable risk factors to make a difference in your future health and well-being. You should do everything in your power to ensure that in your golden years you will be able to climb a mountain with your loved one to watch a sunset, impulsively jump on a bike and go on a bike ride with your kids or partner, or go on a walk with a favorite friend.

Your physical activity and mental possibilities in your future are limitless—if you take good care of your body now. Your goal should be to have a balance of spirit, mind, and body.

Today, your mission should be to do a health survey: a 100,000 mile road check, to ensure that in your future you can fully enjoy every moment. Empowered with well-earned robust health to climb any mountain, swim any sea, and sore like an eagle. Take action now in order to celebrate your health and well-being through your entire life.

Let's get started today. Prevention and health maintenance are your gifts to yourself and your family for a healthy, energized today and a fabulous tomorrow. Preventive lifestyle choices increase your joy of living and diminish your fear of dying of diseases that are preventable. You are in control of your quality of life. Make healthy lifestyle choices today and live a robust life for all of your years.

Your Personal Health Survey: Balancing Spirit, Mind, and Body Category

	YES	NO	New Goals

Spirit

- You are happy most of the time ____ ____
- You have a positive attitude most of the time ____ ____
- You have a social support system of family and friends ____ ____
- You cope well with most situations ____ ____
- You laugh or smile at least once daily ____ ____
- You believe in God ____ ____
- You control your temper most of the time ____ ____
- You feel liked or loved by others ____ ____
- You feel connected to family and friends and engaged in life ____ ____
- You have an overall good sense of well-being ____ ____

Spirit Total ____ ____

Mind

- You have a pet ____ ____
- You read, write, or work on a mental activity daily ____ ____
- You have a hobby or enjoy art or music ____ ____
- You enjoy movies, game shows, or games ____ ____
- You get 7–8 hours of sleep per night ____ ____
- You get 10 minutes of fresh air daily ____ ____
- You have 15 minutes of "you" time everyday to indulge and enjoy yourself or to just rest, restore, and rejuvenate ____ ____
- You avoid people who give you side effects (emotionally/physically) ____ ____

Mind Total ____ ____

Body

- You maintain a healthy weight ____ ____
- You do daily exercises for 30 minutes ____ ____
- You do toning: lifting light weights, increasing repetition several times weekly ____ ____
- You eat a nutritious, balanced diet (low calorie, low fat, sugars, salts) most days ____ ____
- You eat 5+ fruits and vegetables daily ____ ____
- You eat 25 grams of fiber most days ____ ____
- Your blood pressure is less than 130/85 mmHg ____ ____
- Your fasting blood sugar is less than 110 mg/dl ____ ____
- Your cholesterol is less than 200 mg/dl; triglycerides less than 150 mg/dl; HDL greater than 45 mg/dl; LDL less than 130 mg/dl (less than 100 mg/dl if you have heart disease or diabetes) ____ ____
- You eat serving-size portions most of the time ____ ____
- You eat breakfast most days ____ ____
- You drink less than 4 oz wine, 12 oz beer, or 1.5 oz spirits per day ____ ____
- You drink less than 12 oz caffeine per day ____ ____
- You do not smoke ____ ____

Body Total ____ ____

Spirit, Mind, Body, Category Grand Total ____ ____

Your Personal Health Survey: Safety, Prevention, and Health Maintenance Category

	YES	NO	New Goals
Safety First			
• You always wear your seatbelt	___	___	
• You wear sunscreen when exposed to the sun	___	___	
• You think of safety first, and wear the necessary safety gear for your activities (sports, work, hobbies, home jobs)	___	___	
• You drive the speed limit	___	___	
• You practice safe sex (against STDs and unwanted pregnancy)	___	___	
• You do not use recreational drugs	___	___	
• You wear sunglasses in the sun	___	___	
• You have smoke alarms (with good batteries)	___	___	
• You have a carbon monoxide detector	___	___	
Safety Total	___	___	
Prevention			
• You are current on your tetanus shot (and flu and pneumonia shots, if warranted)	___	___	
• You take one daily multivitamin	___	___	
• You take an aspirin (81 mg) per day (if okayed by doctor)	___	___	
• You take or eat 1200+ mg (1500 mg if postmenopausal) of calcium with vitamin D daily	___	___	
• You take your prescribed medications	___	___	
• You have told your doctor about all items you are taking or using including prescription drugs, vitamins, aspirin, herbal remedies, over-the-counter drugs, creams, etc.	___	___	
Prevention Total	___	___	
Health Maintenance			
• You get physicals every one to two years (including blood pressure, weight, and height)	___	___	
• You get paps and pelvics every one to three years	___	___	
• You get a mammogram; if age 40–49 every one to two years, yearly if you are 50+	___	___	
• You do monthly self breast exams	___	___	
• You have gotten a screening bone density test at age 65 (or sooner if family osteoporosis history, history of fracture, or low calcium intake warrants it)	___	___	
• You see your eye doctor and dentist every six months to one year	___	___	
• You have gotten a screening colon study at age 50 (age 40 if high risk factors)	___	___	
• You have gotten screening labs including cholesterol, LDL, HDL, triglycerides, and blood sugar (and thyroid at age 50)	___	___	
Health Maintenance Total	___	___	
Safety, Prevention, and Health Maintenance Category Grand Total	___	___	

Your Results

Now is the exciting time to grade yourself and see what opportunities you have to add years to your life and quality to your years.

Your grade for the total of spirit, mind, and body category:

A=27–32 yes   **B**=20–26 yes   **C**=13–19 yes   **D**=8–12 yes   **F**=0–7 yes

_____**(A)**   **A**wesome! All right, congratulations. You are making great health choices, keep up the good work.

_____**(B)**   **B**etter tune up (you could do better). Key in on the areas to improve now. List your new goals and reassess your success in 21 days.

_____**(C)**   **C**ritical changes could be made now to change your future. List your new goals and reassess your success in 21 days.

_____**(D)**   **D**octor needs to be called today for an appointment. Key in on your most critical areas to list new goals and reassess your success in 21 days.

_____**(F)**   **F**orget your 401K, pension plan, and retirement funds that you are working and saving for—you won't be needing them unless you start taking better care of yourself. Key in on your most critical areas to list new goals. Ask your doctor and a friend to help keep you motivated. Reassess your success in 21 days.

Your grade for the total of safety, prevention, and health maintenance category:

A=20–23 yes   **B**=16–19 yes   **C**=10–15 yes   **D**=5–9 yes   **F**=0–4 yes

_____**(A)**   **A**wesome! All right, congratulations. You are making great health choices, keep up the good work.

_____**(B)**   **B**etter tune up (you could do better). Key in on the areas to improve now. List your new goals and reassess your success in 21 days.

_____**(C)**   **C**ritical changes could be made now to change your future. List your new goals and reassess your success in 21 days.

_____**(D)**   **D**octor needs to be called today for an appointment. Key in on your most critical areas to list new goals and reassess your success in 21 days.

_____**(F)**   **F**orget your 401K, pension plan, and retirement funds that you are working and saving for—you won't be needing them unless you start taking better care of yourself. Key in on your most critical areas to list new goals. Ask your doctor and a friend to help keep you motivated. Reassess your success in 21 days.

You can grade yourself for each category of spirit, mind, body, safety, prevention, and health maintenance. Look at each category for ways to improve your grade with your new goals. Make healthy lifestyle choices daily for 21 days by using the information in the following chapters, then take the survey again. You can change your future health through the small adjustments you make today. You can be refreshed, restored, and rejuvenated in your spirit, mind, and body.

How exciting for you to now embrace your health and well-being, and look forward to the wonderful things that you can do right now and in your future to add years to your life, and quality to your years. Take charge of your life and your health and be your personal best.

Your Personal Health Survey (21-Day Reassessment): Balancing Spirit, Mind, and Body Category

	YES	NO	New Goals

Spirit
- You are happy most of the time ____ ____
- You have a positive attitude most of the time ____ ____
- You have a social support system of family and friends ____ ____
- You cope well with most situations ____ ____
- You laugh or smile at least once daily ____ ____
- You believe in God ____ ____
- You control your temper most of the time ____ ____
- You feel liked or loved by others ____ ____
- You feel connected to family and friends and engaged in life ____ ____
- You have an overall good sense of well-being ____ ____

Spirit Total ____ ____

Mind
- You have a pet ____ ____
- You read, write, or work on a mental activity daily ____ ____
- You have a hobby or enjoy art or music ____ ____
- You enjoy movies, game shows, or games ____ ____
- You get 7–8 hours of sleep per night ____ ____
- You get 10 minutes of fresh air daily ____ ____
- You have 15 minutes of "you" time everyday to indulge and enjoy yourself or to just rest, restore, and rejuvenate ____ ____
- You avoid people who give you side effects (emotionally/physically) ____ ____

Mind Total ____ ____

Body
- You maintain a healthy weight ____ ____
- You do daily exercises 30 minutes ____ ____
- You do toning: lifting light weights, increasing repetition several times weekly ____ ____
- You eat a nutritious, balanced diet (low calorie, low fat, sugars, salts) most days ____ ____
- You eat 5+ fruits and vegetables daily ____ ____
- You eat 25 grams of fiber most days ____ ____
- Your blood pressure is less than 130/85 mmHg ____ ____
- Your fasting blood sugar is less than 110 mg/dl ____ ____
- Your cholesterol is less than 200 mg/dl; triglycerides less than 150 mg/dl; HDL greater than 45 mg/dl; LDL less than 130 mg/dl (less than 100 mg/dl if you have heart disease or diabetes) ____ ____
- You eat serving size portions most of the time ____ ____
- You eat breakfast most days ____ ____
- You drink less than 4 oz wine, 12 oz beer, or 1.5 oz spirits per day ____ ____
- You drink less than 12 oz caffeine per day ____ ____
- You do not smoke ____ ____

Body Total ____ ____

Spirit, Mind, Body, Category Grand Total ____ ____

Your Personal Health Survey (21-Day Reassessment): Safety, Prevention, and Health Maintenance Category

Safety First	YES	NO	New Goals
• You always wear your seatbelt	___	___	
• You wear sunscreen when exposed to the sun	___	___	
• You think of safety first, and wear the necessary safety gear for your activities (sports, work, hobbies, home jobs)	___	___	
• You drive the speed limit	___	___	
• You practice safe sex (against STDs and unwanted pregnancy)	___	___	
• You do not use recreational drugs	___	___	
• You wear sunglasses in the sun	___	___	
• You have smoke alarms (with good batteries)	___	___	
• You have a carbon monoxide detector	___	___	
Safety Total	___	___	

Prevention			
• You are current on your tetanus shot (and flu and pneumonia shots, if warranted)	___	___	
• You take one daily multivitamin	___	___	
• You take an aspirin (81 mg) per day (if okayed by doctor)	___	___	
• You take or eat 1200+ mg (1500 mg if postmenopausal) of calcium with vitamin D daily	___	___	
• You take your prescribed medications	___	___	
• You have told your doctor about all items you are taking or using including prescription drugs, vitamins, aspirin, herbal remedies, over-the-counter drugs, creams, etc.	___	___	
Prevention Total	___	___	

Health Maintenance			
• You get physicals every one to two years (including blood pressure, weight, and height)	___	___	
• You get paps and pelvics every one to three years	___	___	
• You get a mammogram; if age 40–49 every one to two years, yearly if you are 50+	___	___	
• You do monthly self breast exams	___	___	
• You have gotten a screening bone density test at age 65 (or sooner if family osteoporosis history, history of fracture, or low calcium intake warrants it)	___	___	
• You see your eye doctor and dentist every six months to one year	___	___	
• You have gotten a screening colon study at age 50 (age 40 if high risk factors)	___	___	
• You have gotten screening labs including cholesterol, LDL, HDL, triglycerides, and blood sugar (and thyroid at age 50)	___	___	
Health Maintenance Total	___	___	
Safety, Prevention, and Health Maintenance Category Grand Total	___	___	

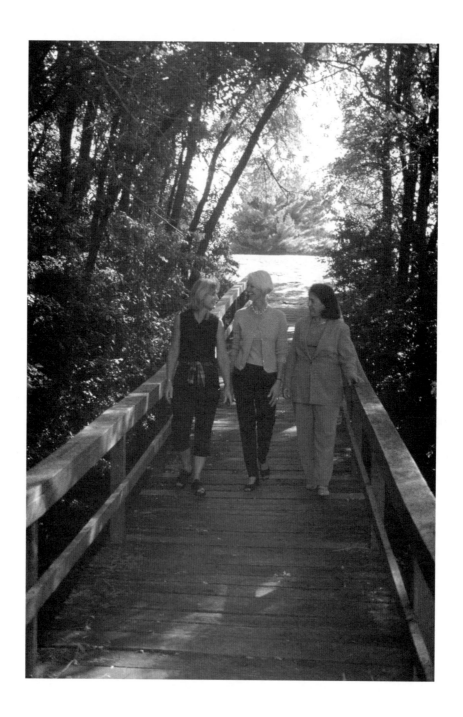

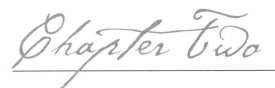

Chapter Two

Staying your best in the future includes having a schedule for health checks. This is an exciting and opportune time for you to embrace your health, improve your well-being, and look forward to a healthy and happy future.

Chapter 2: Empowering Yourself
Staying Your Best

In the chapter "Preventive Health Maintenance," you were able to set new goals of success for yourself in order to add years to your life, and quality to your years. This is an exciting and opportune time for you to embrace your health, improve your well-being, and look forward to a healthy and happy future.

Now is the time to start to take charge of your life and your health and become your personal best. In order for you to stay your best, you need to plan for your future with planned **Health Maintenance Guidelines**; staying your best in the future means having a schedule for health checks. Staying your best also means that you keep your own personal **Health Maintenance Chart** that summarizes your personal health issues, exam/test results, medicines being taken, and family history. It is important to be as accurate as possible about your family history because certain diseases are genetic; you may need early or more aggressive screening for the diseases listed for family members. It is also a good idea to bring your health maintenance chart to your health exams, so you can review with your doctor the tests you may need, or the lifestyle changes you can make to improve your overall well-being.

Take the time now to review the "Staying Your Best: **Health Maintenance Guidelines**" and see what you need to do in order to stay your best. Also complete the **Health Maintenance Chart** and evaluate where you and your doctor can partner together to keep you strong and healthy. In the back of this book you will find duplicates of the **Health Maintenance Guidelines** and the **Health Maintenance Chart** you can cut out; it is a good idea to keep your **Health Maintenance Guidelines** and your **Health Maintenance Chart** together in a conveniently located file, so you can add any changes in your life to these charts, and take them with you to your physical exams.

Congratulations on taking charge of your health and being your best now and in the future!

Staying Your Best: Health Maintenance Guidelines*

	30–39 years	40–49 years	50+ years
Physical Exam	Every 3–5 years	Every 2–3 years	Every 1–2 years
Height	Every 3–5 years	Every 2–3 years	Every 1–2 years
Weight	Every 3–5 years	Every 2–3 years	Every 1–2 years
Eyes	Every 1–2 years	Every 1–2 years	Every 1–2 years
Teeth	Every 6 months	Every 6 months	Every 6 months
Hearing	Age 60 (screen)		
Skin (self exam)	Monthly	Monthly	Monthly
Skin (doctor exam)	Yearly	Yearly	Yearly
Bones		Early screen if history (HX) of hysterectomy, family HX of osteoporosis, adult HX of fracures or low calcium intake or absporption	At least one screening bone density if postmenopausal
Heart*			
Blood Pressure	Every 2–3 years	Every 1–2 years	Every year
Cholesterol	Every 5 years	Every 3–5 years	Once, then every 2–3 years
LDL	Every 5 years	Every 3–5 years	Once, then every 2–3 years
Triglycerides	Every 5 years	Every 3–5 years	Once, then every 2–3 years
HDL	Every 5 years	Every 3–5 years	Once, then every 2–3 years
Diabetes*			
Blood Sugars	Every 3–5 years	Every 3–5 years	Once, then every 3 years (sooner if needed)
Shots			
Tetanus/Diptheria	Every 10 years	Every 10 years	Every 10 years
Influenza	If needed	If needed	Yearly
Pneumonia	If needed	If needed	Once at age 65
Breast			
(self exam)	Monthly	Monthly	Monthly
(clinical exam)	Yearly	Yearly	Yearly
Mammogram	Screen if family history	Every 1–2 yrs	Every year
PAP: cervical**	Every 1–3 years if three in a row are normal	Every 1–3 years if three in a row are normal	Every 1–3 years if always normal
Pelvic (vulvar, vagina, uterus, ovaries)	Every 1–3 years	Every 1–3 years	Every 1–3 years
Thyroid/TSH*	If symptomatic	If symptomatic	Once, then if symptomatic
CBC/UA* (anemia, bladder, kidney screen)	If symptomatic	Once, then if symptomatic	Once, then every 3 years
Colon			
Digital Rectal Exam	If symptomatic	If symptomatic	Yearly
Guaiac/Hemocult	If symptomatic	If symptomatic	Yearly
Flex sig/Barium Enema (BE)	If symptomatic	If symptomatic	Every 3–5 years with BE every 5–10 years
Colonoscopy	If symptomatic, or if increased risk then screening colonoscopy	If symptomatic, or if increased risk then screening colonoscopy	Every 5–10 years. If increased risk or history of polyps, then more frequently (3–5 years)

**For all labs and tests: if any are abnormal, or you have a disease state involving above, labs may need to be checked more frequently.

**Yearly pap if on birth control pill. If hysterectomy for cancer, abnormal cells, or for reasons unknown, then per doctor's orders.

© 2002 Dr. Robin Hartley

On the following page is your **Health Maintenance Chart**. Below is an explanation of terms used on the chart, and how to fill out each section of the chart. This form is the same (or very similar) to the type of form your doctor fills out about you. Taking charge of your physical health includes taking charge of your medical history; make sure you are informed about your past and present medical condition. We have all gone to our doctor's office and wondered what they are writing on those charts—now you will know, and will be able to go to the doctor with your information ready.

Health Maintenance Chart Instructions

Section 1:
Fill in today's date, as well as your name, date of birth, and marital status. **SBE Prophylaxis** refers to whether or not you need an antibiotic before dental work (your doctor can fill in this part).

Section 2:
The Allergies section is where you list all of your allergies, including any allergies to medications or environment. (Ex. Penicillin or ragweed).

Section 3:
PM HX stands for past medical history. In this section you can include any significant medical health history. This could include such items as: pneumonia, mononucleosis, high blood pressure, fractures, diabetes, etc.

Section 4:
P SURG/HOSPITALIZATION is the section where you list any surgical procedures (in- or outpatient), and any hospitalizations you have had.

Section 5:
FAMILY HX is the section for family medical history; include information on whether or not the family members listed are living, and what major medical conditions they have/had. **MGM** represents maternal grandmother, **PGM** represents paternal grandmother, **MGF** represents maternal grandfather, and **PGF** represents paternal grandfather. This section is very important for you because it shows what diseases may be in your genetic makeup. (Ex. If you have three blood relatives who have/have had diabetes, you may want to be checked routinely for diabetes.)

Section 6:
CHRONIC MEDS is where you list any medications or over-the-counter products you take on a regular basis. (Ex. Calcium, multivitamin, insulin, blood pressure medicine and dosage.)

Section 7:
SOC HX is the section where you record your social history. **G** represents the number of pregnancies you have had, **P** represents the number of children you have had. Also in this section, list the types of contraception you have used/are using, what your occupation is, if you are a smoker (**TOB**) and how much you smoke per day, how many cups of coffee (or other caffeine) you consume per day, how many alcoholic drinks you consume per day, whether or not you have a balanced diet, what type of/how much exercising you do, and whether or not you use your seatbelt. You should also record whether or not you have had a tetanus shot as an adult, and the other immunizations you have had/may need. If you are not sure of your immunization status, your doctor will refer to your immunization form for more information. You may also discuss with your doctor which over-the-counter (**OTC**) drugs you are taking, your sexual behavior (monogamous, abstinent, etc.), if you own/use guns, your helmet use (for bicycles or motorcycles), whether or not you wear sunscreen, if you are careful to regulate your water heater temperature, and if you have working smoke and carbon monoxide (**CO**) alarms.

Section 8:
EXAM is the section where you can record the date and results of your last blood pressure (**BP**) check, weight check, height measurement, pap smear, cholesterol check, thyroid stimulating hormone (**TSH**) check, stool occult blood test (**OB**), flex sigmoidoscopy (**Flex Sig**)/barium enema (**BE**), chest X-ray (**CXR**), mammogram, self breast exam, bone density test, and colonoscopy. In this section, you can also record if you are taking a calcium supplement, and if your diet, exercise, and fiber intake are at exceptable levels. In the blank lines you can add any other health-related topics you think you should be monitoring. This section is separated into eight columns—one column per year; so, you can use one chart to monitor your health for eight years.

Section 9:
Advanced Directives refers to what type of care you would like to have if you become unable to make a medical decision (Ex. if you are in a coma). In this section you can also record on what date the advanced directives were last discussed with/received by your doctor, if you have a living will, if someone has durable power of attorney for your health care, and if you are an organ donor.

Health Maintenance Chart

Date __/__/___

Name _____

Date of Birth __/__/___

Status: Married ☐   Single ☐   Divorced ☐   Widowed ☐

SBE Prophylaxis: Yes ☐   No ☐

Allergies _____
_____
_____
_____
_____

PM HX:

P SURG/HOSPITALIZATION _____
_____
_____
_____
_____

FAMILY HX _____

Mother _____

Father _____

MGM _____ PGM _____

MGF _____ PGF _____

Siblings _____
_____
_____

Children _____
_____
_____

Extended _____

SOC HX: G__ P__ Contraception _____

Occupation _____

TOB _____

Coffee: Cups/day___ Other caffeine _____

Alcohol _____ Drinks/day _____

Diet _____

Exercise _____

Seat belt use: Yes ☐ No ☐

Immunizations: ☐ See Immunization Form _____

Discussed: OTC Drug ☐   Sex Behavior ☐   Guns ☐

Helmets ☐   Sunscreen ☐   Water Heater Temp ☐

Smoke Alarm ☐

CO Alarm ☐ _____

CHRONIC MEDS:

EXAM:

Date/Results								
BP								
Weight								
Height								
Pap Smear								
Cholesterol								
TSH								
Colonoscopy								
Stool OB								
Flex Sig/BE								
CXR								
Mammogram								
Calcium Supp.								
Diet/Exer/Fiber								
Self Breast Exam								
Bone Density								

Advanced Directives: Yes ☐ No ☐   Date Discussed __/__/___   Received ☐   Living Will ☐

Durable Power of Attorney for Health Care ☐   Organ Donor Yes ☐ No ☐

© 2002 Dr. Robin Hartley

Note: You should call your insurance company and speak to your doctor to verify your insurance coverage for the tests and labs included in the Health Maintenance Guidelines because this is an aggressive prevention/health maintenance plan; there may be some items that your insurance will cover only at a certain age or on a certain schedule. If you are at high risk and your insurance company will not pay for the above exams, you may consider working out a payment plan for your tests and/or procedures.

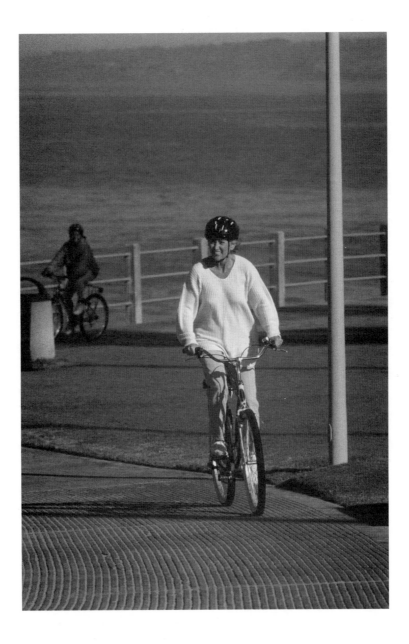

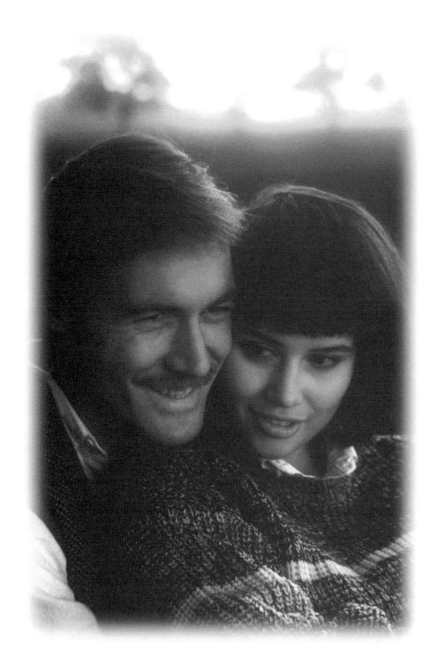

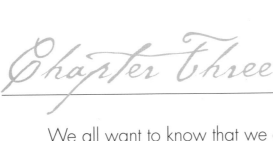

Chapter Three

We all want to know that we are loved and appreciated and that our life matters. We crave that warm smile and loving glance that says "I would marry you all over again if given the chance."

Chapter 3: Romance Me! With a Warm Embrace

"It can't be 5:30 a.m. already," Karen said to herself as she was abruptly awakened by her alarm. It must be God's joke that there are two 5:30s in one day. It had been such a short night: listening to make sure that the car driven by their newly licensed 16-year-old had rolled into the garage by curfew, trying to turn her brain off from the day's "To Do" list, remembering all of the things she should have done, thinking of things she should have said (or shouldn't have said), and mentally making tomorrow's "To Do" list.

As she was lying in bed, the endless night continuing, Karen noticed her heart seemed to be pounding, then racing—was it beating too fast? Was her heart going to leap right out of her chest? Couldn't Mitch wake up for just a second to take her pulse to see if he thought it was racing? Could this be stress or was it a heart attack? Yes, the clock really did say 5:30 a.m. It was time to get up. "Sleep deprivation doesn't kill people, does it?" Karen thinks, trying to shake off her sleepiness. "Get up, everyone is depending on you. You have to keep going in order to keep everyone else going."

After a quick walk outside and a brief shower, it is time to get the kids up, dressed, breakfasted, and on the right bus going to the right school (harder than one might think with several multi-aged kids going to different schools). Then, Karen breaks all land speed records to get to work and not be too late— but she is already late, so it is all relative.

Once at work, Karen starts climbing the mountain of work on top of her desk. Karen has no time for lunch; her afternoon is spent on the stack of work on her desk, tossing folders, notes and messages off the top as she continues her descent down the paper mountain. Now it is 5:30 p.m.—5:30 again?! Karen leaves the remaining work on her desk, now only a foot hill. She will save the rest for tomorrow.

On the way home, Karen drives through the dry cleaning pickup and gets milk at the convenience store. Once home, she throws in a few loads of laundry while making dinner. Dinner time is supposed to be quality family time, *so sit down now!* After cleaning up the kitchen, it is off to the kid's sport practices, school events, and church activities, and back home just in time to help her youngest with his homework. After all the screaming, yelling, and crying (and that's on Karen's part), the homework is done and it is

Now, it is time for bedtime stories—Karen glances at her watch and realizes it's too late. Sorry, not tonight kids. Was that the dryer bell? Karen sighs and decides the laundry can wait until tomorrow. The home is finally quiet and the kids are at least in their beds—although not asleep, and the kitchen is as clean as it gets.

Finally, Karen has a few minutes of peace and quiet to herself. She flops into bed to enjoy one self-indulgent moment to relax by picking up the magazine that has been at her bedside collecting dust (*add dusting to tomorrow's "To Do" list*). Cozy in bed, smiling to herself that another full day of tasks has been accomplished, Karen is ready for that much-earned sleep. And here comes Mitch, entering the bedroom looking for the best sex of his life. Mitch doesn't realize that Karen has spent her last ounce of energy between the kids, work, and home. Karen had nothing left to give.

Sound familiar? You give so much of your day, there is nothing left to give to each other at the day's end. Because you are often running on empty at the day's end, during the day you need to rediscover the art of holding each other, giving a loving glance, or a soft gentle squeeze to a shoulder. Relearn how to hold your hand in his, share a quick kiss, or experience a warm embrace; they are all things that only take a second, but last in your heart all day long.

We all want to know we are loved and appreciated and that our life matters. We crave that warm smile and loving glance that says "I would marry you all over again if given the chance." These simple, loving things are satisfying and fulfilling. These kinds of gestures of intimacy mean more to most women than any single act of intercourse. A hug does not need to lead to sexual completion. For some, it is difficult to see there is a separation between touching and intercourse.

A hug can be—in and of itself—a warm, selfless gesture. When you hug each other, you are holding onto each other for a brief moment in time, keeping each other safe and protected from the world. With a hug, your souls melt together, your hearts are afire, and your spirits are intertwined. It is as if time stands still, and all is well. Your shared hug has given you empowerment, and has reenergized you. The gentle release from the hug gives you the loving lift to carry you through your day with renewed energy, with your soul now restored until you can be together again.

As a woman, it is often hard to give loving looks and brief touches to your partner because these innocent gestures are seen as the green light to something more. What you are trying to say is "I love you" and "I am glad you are here sharing my world with me." What he hears is "Tonight is my lucky night; she is finally in the mood." Sometimes women revert into their mother role, worker role, or too-busy mode trying not to look at their spouse in the "wrong" way. Often you remain in neutral with your body language and emotions, so you won't give the wrong signal—because as far as you are concerned, tonight is *not* the night! All you really want tonight is a warm embracing hug that says "I love you, you're a great Mom and wife, and you are doing a great job." And if the fantasy were to continue, he would say "Why don't you take a nice long bubble bath? And I'll draw it up for you." The evening would end with your climbing into bed early after he has given you a back massage.

If it were up to some men, they would like to have intercourse five out of seven nights a week. Men say they are happier when they have sex more often. Women, on the other hand, feel that if they are more spiritually connected with their partner, maybe then they will want sex more often. Most women would be satisfied with intercourse one out of ten nights—if it is of quality. If your relationship is more intimate with daily warm embraces, loving kisses, and "I love you" spoken with a meaningful glance, then one out of 30 nights may be satisfactory.

Most women want the intimacy. Most men want to cut to the chase. Women love the romance of the relationship first, and then they are ready for the adventure. "Romance me!" you say. Women want the intimacy of lifelong courting. Things like love notes scribbled on the "To Do" list, the unexpected "I'm thinking of you" card, phone calls, flowers, candlelight, and wine and dinner get our hearts on fire. We just want to know our partners are inside our souls breathing a breath of life into our spirit. Once our souls connect and we are breathing the same breath, then our bodies can be together in a sweet serenade.

Then Again...

The stage was set. Ann had prepared a rose petal trail from the front door to the bedroom for when Jason arrived home. Ann had placed scented candles to line the hallway to their bedroom giving off an inviting glow. Their life was turning out okay. Jason had a good job. The kids were grown and gone. It was just them now. It was time to get their life back. Time just for "us" and time to rediscover each other. Jason arrived home to a George Benson CD filling the air with soft melodies. Ann had put on her slinkiest lingerie and the romantic kissing and touching between Ann and Jason began. The passion escalated and the kissing became more intense. Then...nothing. They had both silently taken their most historically successful sex positions. After 18 years of marriage, they knew what worked, and they did not want to change a thing. But, nothing was happening for Jason. At first, Ann felt sorry for Jason. Then Ann's thoughts turned to herself. Could *she* be the reason Jason couldn't perform tonight? Jason had said that the extra 20 pounds Ann had gained over the years didn't really matter—but it *must*. Or, was it something she had done? Was it that Jason just wasn't interested anymore? There must be somebody else. Jason, unable to perform and feeling frustrated and helpless, retreated to the den to be with his mistress—the computer. With the simple touch of a key, he could escape from the reality of impotency with aging. Ann felt cold, rejected, and alone in the bed not sure what to do or what to think.

How do you keep the passion alive? How do you keep your hearts afire for a lifetime? It is easier than you think. You can't put your life on hold, or on auto pilot, and think that when the kids are grown, when your jobs are stable, when your relationships with family and friends are in good order, then you will have the time and energy to give to your partner. Just as you must eat food daily to fuel your body for energy, you must give time and effort daily to fuel your relationship with your partner—to keep your love life alive and keep the fires burning.

And remember—your partner can't read your mind. You will need to tell him what you desire—or better yet, *you* be the instigator by taking your relationship to the next level. Fuel the love fire, every day, in order to be able to celebrate your golden years together. Consider the suggestions on the following page as "gold nuggets" of investment to ensure your enjoyment of the riches of love in your golden years together.

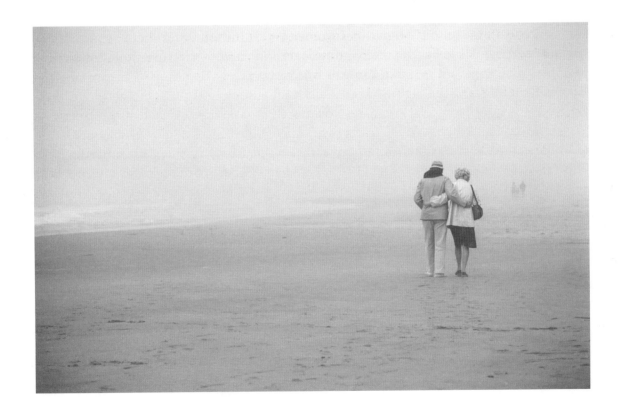

Worth Shaving Your Legs For...
Gold nuggets to enhance the richness of your love.

- Buy a scented candle for the bedroom. Candlelight glow makes a woman feel young and beautiful.

- Turn the TV off in the bedroom. Your bodies deserve your full attention. A quickie during halftime does not count.

- Put away the Playboy magazines. We shouldn't have to compete and feel defeated before even getting started.

- Give one single, long-stem rose unexpectedly. This softens the hardest of days.

- Say I love you—expecting nothing in return.

- Give a warm embrace in the a.m. to start the day out right, knowing you have given each other a love shield to hold in front of you to ricochet off anything that comes your way.

- Write a sweet love note and put it into a lunch bag or briefcase.

- Give an unexpected mid-afternoon phone call just to say "thinking of you and miss you."

- Send an e-mail saying "I can't wait to see you tonight."

- Say something really nice about your partner to a friend loud enough so your partner can hear you.

- Explain to him that you want him to talk to you. Ask him to share his most intimate feelings and secrets with you. Let him know he can trust you with his soul.

- Ask him to just listen to you and let you unload about a situation—you don't need him to try and "fix" it. Let him know you just want him to hold your hand—touch it, squeeze it. Let him know that these gestures say that he is your touchstone and his touch can reenergize you.

- Draw a warm bubble bath for your partner after a trying day just to say "I care."

- Give each other back massages. Gentle, caressing hands send heat to our hearts.

- Pamper each other's feet. A little baby oil and massage applied to pressure points of the foot soles fills the soul with tender joy.

- Give special treatment to the scalp. A gentle scalp massage and shampoo with loving hands relaxes anyone. Combing each other's hair also feels wonderful.

- Spend a weekend alone. Sometimes you have to love someone enough to set them free to be by themselves for the weekend; then, when they come back, they are remotivated and reinspired to be with you. It's like the quote says "If you love somebody, set them free. If they return, they were always yours. If they don't, they never were."

- Give them the gift of music. Buy their favorite CD and have it playing for them when they arrive home.

- Have breakfast in bed. Favorite foods and morning newspaper = pamper.

- Give them a kiss. Quick, or long and passionate to tell them they still have what it takes to turn you on.

- Look into each other's eyes when talking. Our eyes give our partner a window passage to our souls.

- Buy a surprise ticket to your partner's favorite sports, musical, or entertainment event.

- Try a new position and let the fantasy begin.

- Use touch. Use ice cubes, a single feather. Be creative with your touch. (No intercourse allowed)

- Rediscover the sense of smell. Cover your partner's eyes with a silk scarf and place their favorite perfume, cologne, or food scents (one at a time) on your finger and have them guess which one they are smelling and what thoughts or memories those scents evoke. Use senses to awaken the spirit.

- Forget your modesty—if just for one night.

- Rediscover the sense of sight. Make the bedroom a place of joy, warmth, and security by using your favorite colors, plants, and furnishings.

- Buy some lingerie that makes you feel special. Let your partner watch you put it on—or take it off!

- Try toys. Not your style? Think again. Slumber Parties Inc. sales are projected to top over 20 million dollars this year. Products range from Wild Cherry flavored Edible Body Butter (that is sugar-free, fat-free, and FDA approved) to massage sets and more. Patty Brisen, the company's founder, has a RN background and feels there is a need for women to be educated about their bodies. Women of all types, shapes, and sizes are enjoying choosing special items for home use at these private parties.

- Watch a movie. Try something that gets your attention: "9 1/2 Weeks" is good for beginners.

- Have the kids stay with their grandparents for the weekend; this gives the two generations a chance to bond.

- Plan a weekend getaway for just you two, even if you have to create a bed and breakfast in your own home.

- Buy each other special jewelry. Every glance gives remembrances of love.

- Make a great dinner. Prepare your favorite foods side-by-side in the kitchen. The aroma will get you sizzling.

- Dinner table. Bring out the china and crystal. (What are you saving it for anyway?) Use actual cloth napkins. Go ahead! They will add to the special ambiance.

- Buy some wine. Splurge on your favorite bottle and enjoy.

- Don't forget dessert. Indulge yourselves in rich decadence. Share the same utensil. Don't worry about the calories, you will burn them off later.

- Walk together daily. Walking gives you the quality time together you have been looking for and allows you to escape from all the bells, buzzers, and beepers of daily life. Walking gives you time to reconnect your thoughts about life while decreasing your risk of osteoporosis, cancer, and heart disease.

- Remember to keep courting each other every day by doing those things that made your relationship unique; visit a special place, give that certain flower, or celebrate a significant holiday.

- Have a date night. One night a week, have a date together to remind yourselves what it was that you found attractive about each other in the beginning, and what made you want to spend your life together. Each date reconfirms that you would marry each other all over again.

- Reinstate your vows whether it is a big affair complete with orchestra and a minister, or just the two of you saying heartfelt words to each other while alone in your bedroom. Recommit yourself to each other.

Invest in love by giving a "gold nugget" of love to your partner today, it will make your life forever rich.

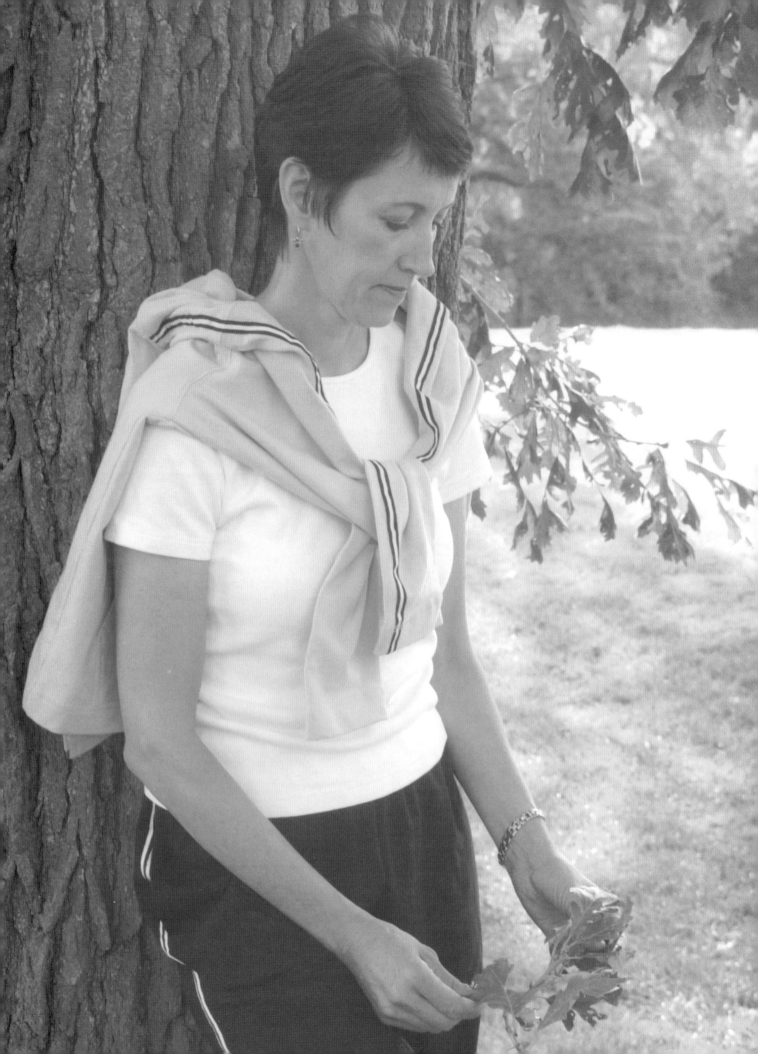

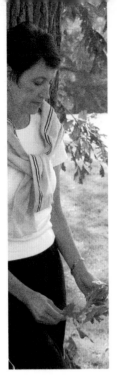

Simplify Your Life

REGAIN CONTROL AND REDISCOVER JOY

Live in the moment you are in this very second. Make the very most of this moment. You will live with the satisfaction of doing the right thing, right now. The past is history; the future is yours by controlling the moment you have now.

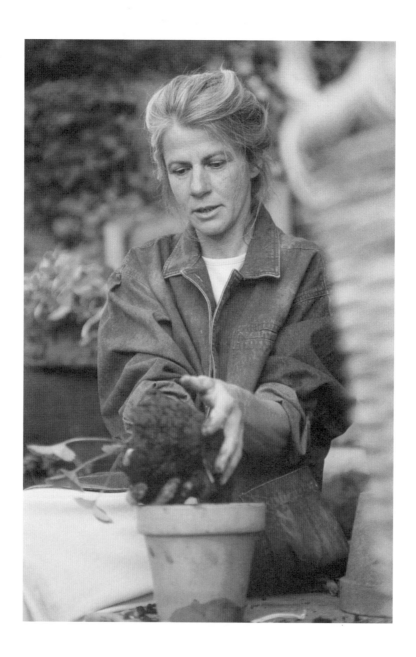

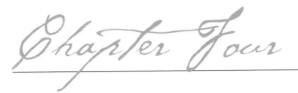

Chapter Four

Instead of carefully selecting your activities, you have become a professional "plate spinner" of life; you're feverishly trying to keep all of your plates spinning on long, thin sticks—so they don't stop spinning and go crashing to the floor in a broken heap.

Chapter 4: *Simplify Your Life Regain Control and Rediscover Joy*

Life is short! Go for the gusto! Be first! Win, win! Let's go! Don't miss out! You won't get a second chance to make a first impression! Hurry up, someone is waiting! Come on! Put your shoes on in the car—we've got to go! There isn't time for a sit-down dinner, let's go through the drive-through and eat in the car on the way to the game! Now isn't that being efficient?!

Sound familiar? Are these the inspirational words that you fuel your mind with to keep your body going through your hectic day? Your endless "To Do" list can make your day seem like a marathon.

Blasting through your busy day of tasks, you race to the mall to find your son shoes for tonight's basketball game. You sprint from store to store—you have 20 minutes before you have to pick up your son after school. You notice the person walking in front of you, thinking to yourself that if they walk any slower they are going to fall over sideways! You just want to shout, "Move out of the way, I'm in a hurry!" Doesn't this person know how busy you are? With the new shoes in hand, you arrive at school with two minutes to spare. Thank goodness you remember you are also supposed to pick up your daughter after school today too. It helps that she is out in front of the school waving her backpack at you and screaming, "Mom!" as you are driving by.

After dropping the kids off at grandma's, you stop by the grocery store to pick up milk and a few other items. You have no time today to be distracted by the "I want" battles in the aisles.

The cart you grab away from the outstretched arms of the lady ahead of you has good working wheels—or so you think—until you notice that one of the wheels is twisted backwards and elevated. You are a pro at dysfunctional carts, so it won't slow you down to balance the tipping tripod cart with your one foot as you race through the aisles.

What a great idea for them to place the milk in the back of the store, so you get to grab a few "necessities" on the way back to the milk! You break your own personal–best time for grocery shopping by reaching the finish line (okay, checkout line) in less than fifteen minutes with $140 worth of goodies. Weren't you just shopping for milk?

At the checkout line you are lucky enough to jockey your cart in front of the lady aiming for "your" spot in line when she hesitates and looks at a magazine cover. (She's the same lady who was going for "your" cart, earlier). Today has been a good day. After all, you made it home with two kids *and* the groceries! At least this time you didn't have to turn the van around halfway home to go back and get the forgotten groceries at the grocery pickup station.

Somehow, you have gotten trapped in the maze of life—racing from one activity to the next, never in control of your path or destination. You tell yourself that the more you get done in the day, the more you can justify your time and be respected for your accomplishments. The more activities you and your family are involved in, the better. Idle hands don't pay the bills or get things done. You feel like you need to justify your existence on this earth with a big check mark on your "To Do" list of life. It is easy to get caught up in the whirlwind of daily activities that have you racing from one task to the next. At the day's end, you feel exhausted, depleted, and somehow empty—despite all of your tasks having been completed.

When tasks are completed successfully, it should make you feel empowered and in control! So why does your life seem so out of control? Probably because it is. You are allowing your daily tasks to dictate who you are and what you do during the day. Instead, you should do activities that reflect who you are.

Instead of carefully selecting your activities, you have become a professional "plate spinner of life" feverishly trying to keep all of your plates spinning on long, thin sticks—so they don't stop spinning and go crashing to the floor in a broken heap. It is as if each one of those plates represents an activity or person in your life that you are attempting to support and nurture—to keep their plate spinning—so they don't go crashing to the floor into a heap of broken hearts or dreams.

Look again at this scenario: the only plate missing is yours! In this fast spinning world of ours, it is easy to get caught up in being the busy plate spinner. You are busy, busy, busy spinning plates, never stopping a minute to enjoy your present surroundings. It is easy to start thinking that because you are a mother, wife, daughter, friend, and/or employee that you are indispensable and everything and everyone depends on you. After all, if not for you, who would keep everyone's plate spinning? Instead of it being a privilege and a pleasure to be a mother, wife, daughter, friend, and/or employee, it becomes a burden. When you allow yourself to escape from your daily tasks (plate spinning) by going on a vacation, you come back with a fresh view and a new attitude. After returning from a vacation, you are rejuvenated with a healthy glow, ready to get back at it—and start your plates spinning again.

Your vacation time is usually the only window of opportunity when you allow yourself to indulge in your spirit, mind, and body. On vacation, your senses become reborn and alive. You allow time for your eyes to see things for the first time or in a different view. You allow time for your nose to smell the wonderful scents of a vanilla candle, fresh-baked cookies, or the tingling salty sea air as you inhale the joys of the world around you. Your ears perk; you hear the thunderous roar of the ocean waves crashing onto the beach, or the merry giggles of children playing at a nearby park. You allow the harmonious symphony of sounds to cascade around you, engulfing and bathing you with peace and a sense of well-being. Even your tastebuds rejoice with pleasure as you indulge in every decadent, delicious morsel of life. On vacation, you reach out to touch your world, and your world eagerly welcomes you back with a warm embracing hug. Sounds wonderful, doesn't it? Life is short, don't wait for a vacation day to start enjoying your life. Your world is waiting for you now!

Take a break from your life; take a step back to look at your world from the outside. That one step back may put you leaps and bounds ahead of anything you had dreamed that you would accomplish in your life.

On vacation, you allow yourself to break the daily habits that hold you as a prisoner trapped in a world of daily self-imposed rituals. Rituals like reading the paper for 20 minutes every morning, drinking three cups of coffee before noon, or watching TV every night. When you step back and critically evaluate your day, you may actually see how your daily rituals are inefficient, unnecessary, or even a road block preventing you from accomplishing your dreams, living a healthy lifestyle, or feeling good about life.

The magic key of getting control back in your life is not to get busier and work harder, but to simplify your life. As for the people in your life for whom you thought you had to keep their plates spinning, do not worry; they can spin their own plate. They are responsible for their own world. By your own example you can show others how to simplify their lives in order to have more abundant lives.

Tips on How to Simplify Your Life

S   **Senses**   Allow your senses of vision, smell, taste, hearing, and touch to be reborn and alive in order to enjoy every morsel of life.

I   **Imagination**   Imagine yourself feeling joyous. Do whatever activities will allow you to arrive at being joyous. Learn a new craft, take a class, complete a degree, try a new sport, or discover a new hobby.

M   **Moment**   Live in the moment you are in this very second. Make the very most of this moment. You will live with the satisfaction of doing the right thing, right now. The past is history; the future is yours by controlling the moment you have now.

P   **Priorities**   List your top five priorities. Your daily activities should reflect and nurture these priorities.

L   **Love**   Allow time to show how much you care to those you care about most. Love makes your life abundant and full of riches.

I   **Invest**   Invest and save enough money for the future, so you don't have to worry about the future—don't forget to live for today, though. Work should be a *part of you, but not who you are.*

F   **Family**   Embrace the joy, the celebrations, and the memories created together. Your memories are your greatest treasure.

Y   **You**   Take care of *you!* Exercise, stretch, eat well, sleep well, and do activities to enrich your spirit, mind, and body. Read a book, take a bubble bath, take a walk through a park. Take care of yourself, so you can feel alive at every moment.

L   **Live**   Live! Release yourself from the mental chains that bind you to habits. Leap out of your chair parked on the curb watching your life parade before you. Jump into your life. Take the scuba class, paint, design a home, go parasailing, hug someone, play with a child, plant a tree.

I   **Indulge**   Indulge daily in a simple pleasure! Eat a piece of chocolate and savor the taste, sit on the deck chair and watch a sunset, walk barefoot in the grass, have a glass of champagne to celebrate your life!

F   **Focus**   Focus on what you are doing and get it done, so you can have more free time.

E   **Enjoy**   Enjoy by eliminating. First, address each issue that arises only once by making a decision or acting on it immediately. Second, learn the joy of giving. Give away your stacks of treasures that you do not really need. Follow these two rules to rid your life of clutter, stacks, "To Do" lists, boxes, and piles.

Regain control and rediscover joy when you simplify your life in order to have a more abundant life!

© 2002 Dr. Robin Hartley

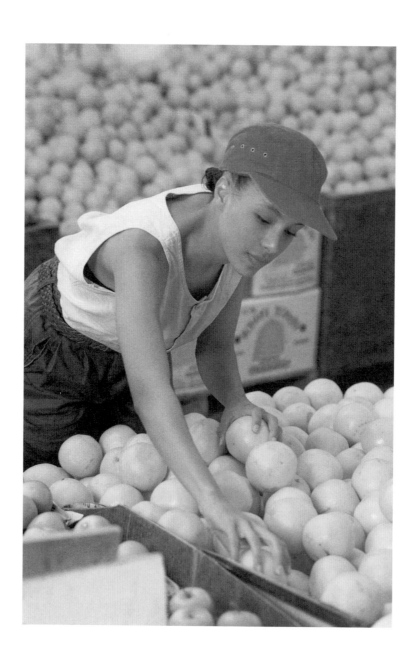

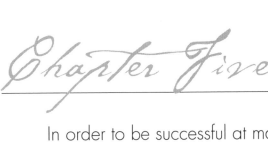

Chapter Five

In order to be successful at making healthier choices, you will need a plan. The Healthzone provides you with such a plan. It is easy to follow, and gives you the power to select the foods that you prefer; it allows you the freedom to enjoy the celebrations in your life.

Chapter 5: Enjoy Your Life
Plan Healthy Living

It feels good to eat healthy foods. When you make healthy choices, you feel you are in control, and you feel better about yourself. "Today is going to be different," you say to yourself. Today you are going to be better about making healthier food choices by watching the salt, sugar, and fat quantities that you consume.

When you woke up today, you had all the best intentions of taking better care of yourself, but the day started out with your running late for work. "Breakfast" ended up being coffee swimming with cream and sugar from the corner convenience store. The cream was for calcium and the sugar and caffeine were to keep you energized. However, by 9:30 a.m. the sugar and caffeine surge was plummeting. Fortunately, a co-worker brought an apple strudel for someone's birthday. You downed the apple strudel guiltlessly (the apple counted for a fruit serving, right?), and you were reenergized until lunch.

You brought a nutritious lunch to work which consisted of yogurt and a banana. But everyone else from the office was going out to the co-worker's birthday lunch. You stood there holding your lifeless brown paper bag and opted to throw it back in the refrigerator and join the birthday celebration.

The lunch was grand—with tasty hors d'oeuvres, a hearty entree, and a wedge of cake topped with a mountain of ice cream.

Everyone was enjoying themselves and telling hilarious stories about one another as you waited for your bill to arrive. You laughed a little too hard at a story and the top button of your pants exploded off and bounced noisily across the tile floor. This sent your co-workers into an uproar of laughter as you sheepishly crawled across the floor to retrieve the evidence of your overindulgence.

Evening arrived and you were full of guilt from overeating during the day, and you were too tired to exercise. Despite being hungry, you chose not to prepare a meal—but, instead, nibbled your way through the evening while you watched television and talked to friends on the phone. You were enticed, intrigued, and tempted as you watched the tantalizing food commercials. By 10:00 p.m. you couldn't stand your hunger any longer; the commercials' persistence had worn down your resistance. You ran to the kitchen and ripped open bags of food to consume them as fast as you could. Maybe tomorrow you could start to take better care of yourself. After all, tomorrow morning was a safe 450 minutes away from today.

As you went to sleep that night, you hoped that sleeping would magically transform your way of thinking about food, and that your eating habits would be at a healthier level by the time you awoke the next day. When you awoke in the morning, nothing had changed. You sank right back into the same old eating habits and lifestyle all over again.

Often, the way you eat is a habit. When you think about it, food is for fuel or energy, period. Food can not fill the voids in your life. Food shouldn't be used to make you feel cared about, provided for, or loved. Food should not be used to get rid of boredom. It can't comfort or console you. Food can't control you, another person, or a situation. You are in control of your food. If you are currently eating to fill the emptiness in your soul, choose instead to be in control by making different choices.

In order to be successful at making healthier choices, you will need a plan. The Healthzone provides you with such a plan. It is easy to follow, and gives you the power to select the foods you prefer. It allows you the freedom to enjoy the celebrations in your life. No foods are forbidden or eliminated on the plan. You will not need to do extreme dieting, buy special foods, or give up your favorite foods. All foods can be a part of a healthy, balanced diet. The Healthzone Plan is based on serving sizes and a version of the food pyramid.

Right now, make the decision to be better to yourself everyday and to enjoy your life! Here are your free benefits for making healthier choices:

Your Rewards for Making Healthy Choices and Your Benefits of Eating Healthier and Exercising

Increased	Decreased Risk of
Energy	Diabetes
Bone density	High blood pressure
Endurance	Heart disease
Endorphins (natural feel good chemicals)	Cholesterol
Self-esteem	Colon cancer
Agility	Breast cancer
Sharpness of mind	Osteoporosis
Weight maintenance	Obesity
Quality of sleep	
Quality of sex	
Joy	
Strength	
Fitness	

Let's Get Started: Your Healthzone Plan

Healthy living and weight maintenance start with a health plan that includes vegetables and fruits as a good foundation. Carbohydrates, proteins, and dairy products are added for nutritional balance. One to two servings of fats and sweets are provided. If you are going to a special celebration, you may need to decrease your carbohydrates or increase your exercise for that day in order to balance your choices. Never eliminate any food category, as your body needs a variety of foods every day for good health and well-being.

Getting your body moving with activities and staying hydrated form the base for your Healthzone Plan. You are only 21 days from being healthier and more energized.

Healthzone Plan: 21 Days to Success

Here is your 21-day plan to healthier living. It is easy to follow. You can cut out the duplicates of the following three pyramid pages from the back of this book and place them in a convenient location. Each pyramid represents one day in the 21-day plan. Each pyramid has boxes that represent the healthy amounts of serving sizes you should have each day for each category.

As you eat a serving of food, do some exercise, or do a positive thought, deed, or action, put a check mark in the box to keep track of your healthy choices. **Your goal is to have most boxes marked off most days.** Each day is a fresh start for a new you. Follow this plan for six days and then take a day off; then, continue the plan the next day. Feel rejuvenated and energized in 21 days. **The secret to your success is to eat a serving size of each of the foods that you select and to keep your body moving!**

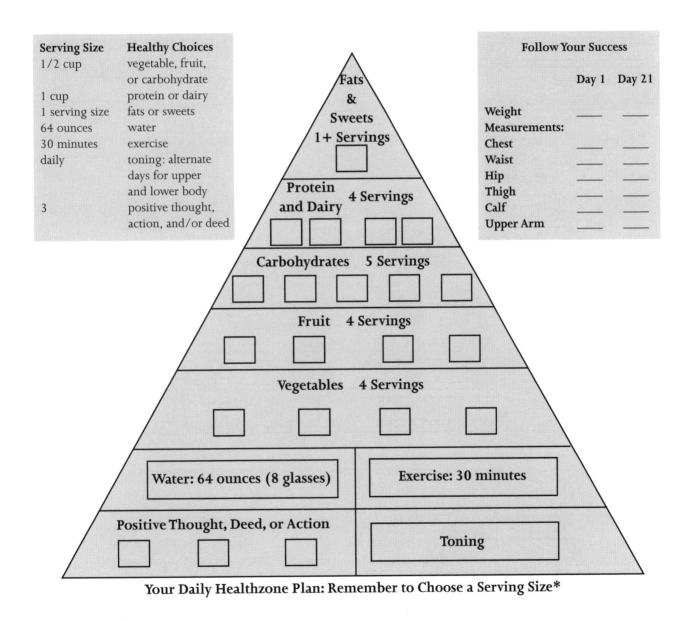

Serving Size	Healthy Choices
1/2 cup	vegetable, fruit, or carbohydrate
1 cup	protein or dairy
1 serving size	fats or sweets
64 ounces	water
30 minutes	exercise
daily	toning: alternate days for upper and lower body
3	positive thought, action, and/or deed

Follow Your Success

	Day 1	Day 21
Weight	____	____
Measurements:		
Chest	____	____
Waist	____	____
Hip	____	____
Thigh	____	____
Calf	____	____
Upper Arm	____	____

Fats & Sweets 1+ Servings

Protein and Dairy 4 Servings

Carbohydrates 5 Servings

Fruit 4 Servings

Vegetables 4 Servings

Water: 64 ounces (8 glasses)   Exercise: 30 minutes

Positive Thought, Deed, or Action   Toning

Your Daily Healthzone Plan: Remember to Choose a Serving Size*

*Pyramid based on a daily calorie intake consisting of 1400 calories a day. See "Daily Serving Sizes Suggested" chart on page 43 to create a Healthzone Plan based on a 1600 or 1800 daily calorie intake.

Food pyramid information adapted with permission from the "Mayo Clinic Healthy Weight Pyramid," © 2001 Mayo Foundation for Medical Education and Research, Rochester, Minnesota

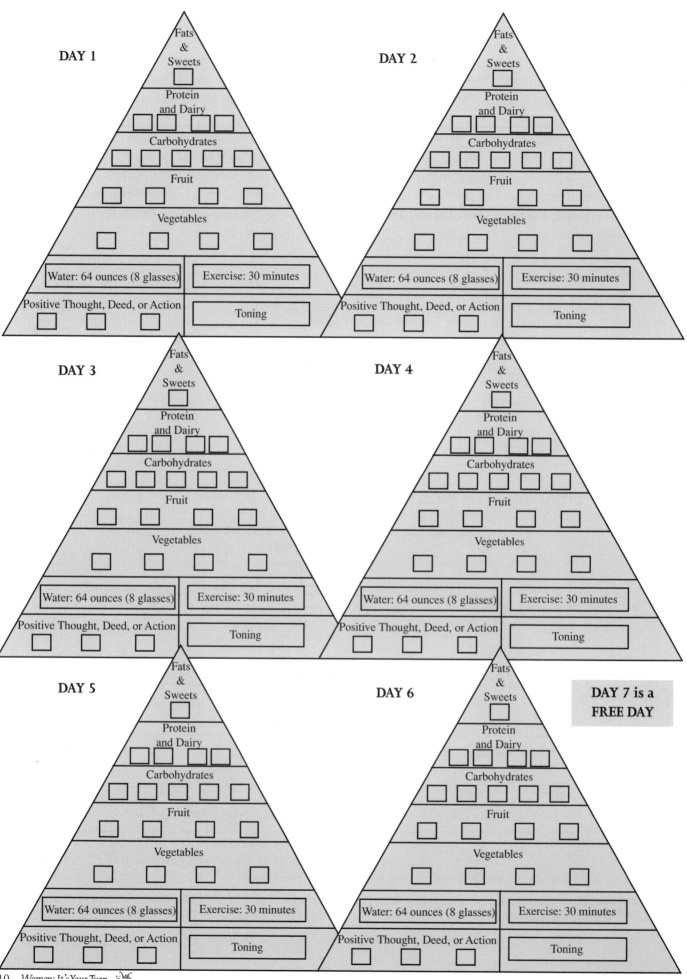

DAY 1

Fats & Sweets

Protein and Dairy

Carbohydrates

Fruit

Vegetables

Water: 64 ounces (8 glasses)

Exercise: 30 minutes

Positive Thought, Deed, or Action

Toning

DAY 2

Fats & Sweets

Protein and Dairy

Carbohydrates

Fruit

Vegetables

Water: 64 ounces (8 glasses)

Exercise: 30 minutes

Positive Thought, Deed, or Action

Toning

DAY 3

Fats & Sweets

Protein and Dairy

Carbohydrates

Fruit

Vegetables

Water: 64 ounces (8 glasses)

Exercise: 30 minutes

Positive Thought, Deed, or Action

Toning

DAY 4

Fats & Sweets

Protein and Dairy

Carbohydrates

Fruit

Vegetables

Water: 64 ounces (8 glasses)

Exercise: 30 minutes

Positive Thought, Deed, or Action

Toning

DAY 5

Fats & Sweets

Protein and Dairy

Carbohydrates

Fruit

Vegetables

Water: 64 ounces (8 glasses)

Exercise: 30 minutes

Positive Thought, Deed, or Action

Toning

DAY 6

Fats & Sweets

Protein and Dairy

Carbohydrates

Fruit

Vegetables

Water: 64 ounces (8 glasses)

Exercise: 30 minutes

Positive Thought, Deed, or Action

Toning

DAY 7 is a FREE DAY

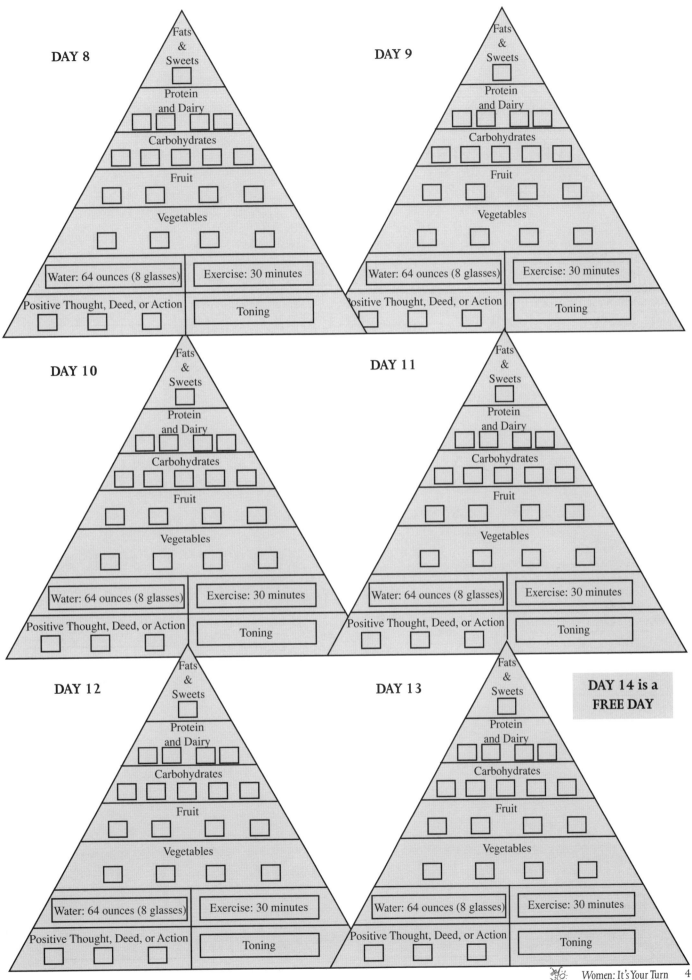

DAY 8

Fats & Sweets

Protein and Dairy

Carbohydrates

Fruit

Vegetables

Water: 64 ounces (8 glasses)

Exercise: 30 minutes

Positive Thought, Deed, or Action

Toning

DAY 9

Fats & Sweets

Protein and Dairy

Carbohydrates

Fruit

Vegetables

Water: 64 ounces (8 glasses)

Exercise: 30 minutes

Positive Thought, Deed, or Action

Toning

DAY 10

Fats & Sweets

Protein and Dairy

Carbohydrates

Fruit

Vegetables

Water: 64 ounces (8 glasses)

Exercise: 30 minutes

Positive Thought, Deed, or Action

Toning

DAY 11

Fats & Sweets

Protein and Dairy

Carbohydrates

Fruit

Vegetables

Water: 64 ounces (8 glasses)

Exercise: 30 minutes

Positive Thought, Deed, or Action

Toning

DAY 12

Fats & Sweets

Protein and Dairy

Carbohydrates

Fruit

Vegetables

Water: 64 ounces (8 glasses)

Exercise: 30 minutes

Positive Thought, Deed, or Action

Toning

DAY 13

Fats & Sweets

Protein and Dairy

Carbohydrates

Fruit

Vegetables

Water: 64 ounces (8 glasses)

Exercise: 30 minutes

Positive Thought, Deed, or Action

Toning

DAY 14 is a FREE DAY

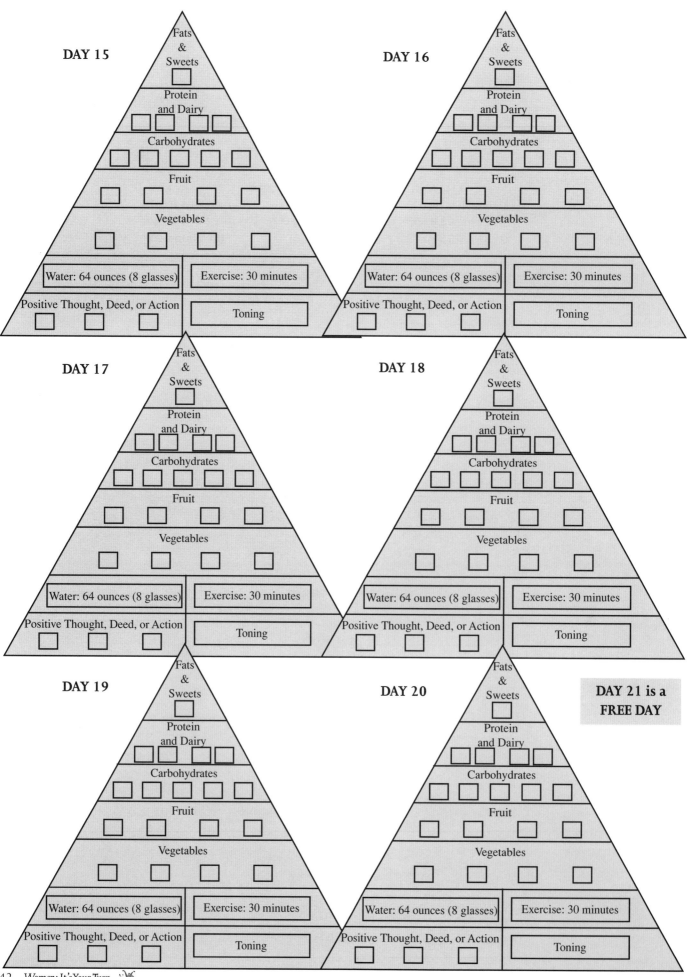

DAY 15

Fats & Sweets

Protein and Dairy

Carbohydrates

Fruit

Vegetables

Water: 64 ounces (8 glasses) | Exercise: 30 minutes

Positive Thought, Deed, or Action | Toning

DAY 16

Fats & Sweets

Protein and Dairy

Carbohydrates

Fruit

Vegetables

Water: 64 ounces (8 glasses) | Exercise: 30 minutes

Positive Thought, Deed, or Action | Toning

DAY 17

Fats & Sweets

Protein and Dairy

Carbohydrates

Fruit

Vegetables

Water: 64 ounces (8 glasses) | Exercise: 30 minutes

Positive Thought, Deed, or Action | Toning

DAY 18

Fats & Sweets

Protein and Dairy

Carbohydrates

Fruit

Vegetables

Water: 64 ounces (8 glasses) | Exercise: 30 minutes

Positive Thought, Deed, or Action | Toning

DAY 19

Fats & Sweets

Protein and Dairy

Carbohydrates

Fruit

Vegetables

Water: 64 ounces (8 glasses) | Exercise: 30 minutes

Positive Thought, Deed, or Action | Toning

DAY 20

Fats & Sweets

Protein and Dairy

Carbohydrates

Fruit

Vegetables

Water: 64 ounces (8 glasses) | Exercise: 30 minutes

Positive Thought, Deed, or Action | Toning

DAY 21 is a FREE DAY

A Quick and Handy Way to Remember Serving Sizes:

One fist = One cup to use for main dish (entree)/protein/dairy/soup

One palm = One-half cup to use for fruit/vegetable/side-dish/carbohydrates

One thumb = Two tablespoons to use for dressing/sauce/gravy/topping

To be good to yourself: drink eight glasses of water a day (64 ounces), and get your body moving with activity.

Daily Serving Sizes Suggested*

Food Category	Activity less than three times a week (1400 calories)	Moderate activity three times a week (1600 calories)	Increased activity five times a week (1800 calories)
Vegetables	4+	5+	5+
Fruit	4+	5+	5+
Carbohydrates	5	6	7
Protein & Dairy	4	5	6
Fats	1+	2+	3+

Notes: Always see a doctor before making any lifestyle or nutritional changes. Increase exercise and decrease calorie intake by 500 calories a day (ex. burn off 200 calories w/exercise and eat 300 less calories of food) in order to lose one to two pounds per week. Caution: Do not just eliminate 500 calories a day from your food intake. Use the body mass index formula to evaluate weight and height: BMI=weight (kg)/height (m2). BMI > 25–29.9=overweight BMI > 30=obese.

*Adapted with permission from the "Mayo Clinic Heathy Weight Pyramid" © 2002 Mayo Foundation for Medical Education and Research, Rochester, MN

Suggested Activities:
(Combine your activities to total 30 minutes or more per day.)

Walking
Bicycling
Dancing
Swimming
Aerobics
Golf
Sweeping
Water Aerobics
Jogging
Racquetball
Tennis
Skiing
Cleaning
Carrying groceries
Rollerblading
Mowing
Gardening
Raking leaves
Shoveling
Stair usage
Polishing the floor/car
Vacuuming

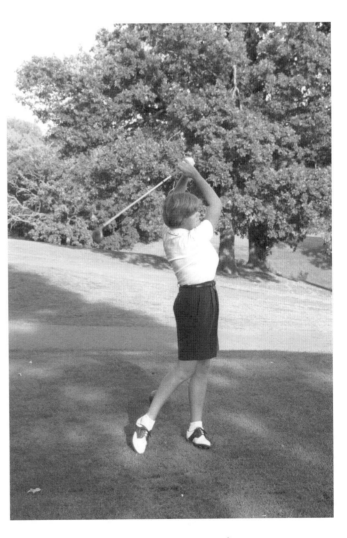

Your Healthzone Plan Guide to Healthy Food Choices*

Vegetables
Serving Size:
Palm full,
1/2 cup raw,
cooked, chopped,
1 cup leafy,
3/4 cup juice

(Fresh, frozen, or steamed are best)

Alfalfa, asparagus, bamboo shoots, bok choy, broccoli, beans, cabbage, chicory, chives, cauliflower, celery, cucumber, egg plant, endive, green beans, garlic, ginger, kale, leeks, lettuce, mushrooms, pepper, parsley, parsnips, radicchio, radishes, sauerkraut, spinach, squash, turnips, turnip greens

Vegetables

With higher levels of carbohydrates* (increased complex sugar)
Beets, brussel sprouts, carrots, collards, okra, onion, rutabaga, rhubarb, peas, tomatoes, artichokes, squash, pumpkin, hominy, water chestnuts, succotash

Vegetables

With the highest levels of carbohydrates*
Corn, potato, sweet potatoes, yams, beans, chick peas, black-eyed peas, soybeans

Fruits
Serving Size:
Palm full,
1/2 cup chopped
or canned,
1 cup fresh,
1 medium-sized,
3/4 cup juice

(Fresh or frozen are best)

< 10 grams of carbohydrates: Blackberries, currants, figs, grapefruit, passion fruit, peaches, plums, tangerines
10–15 grams of carbohydrates: Apricots, avocado, cantaloupe, cherries, cranberries, guava, kiwis, mandarin oranges, mulberries, raspberries, strawberries, watermelon
15–20 grams of carbohydrates: Gooseberries, grapes, honeydew, nectarine, oranges, pineapple
20–25 grams of carbohydrates: Apples, blueberries
> 25 grams of carbohydrates: Banana, boysenberries, dates, elderberries, dried figs, mangoes, papayas, pears, raisins, dried prunes

*Carbohydrates
Serving Size:
1/2 cup rice,
1 slice bread,
1/2 bun, bagel, muffin

Whole grain bread, whole wheat, rye, bran, oat, or barley products; brown, long-grain rice, whole pasta, cereal, wheat or spinach pastas, oatmeal, ricecakes, melba toast, English muffins, tortillas, waffles, pitas, cereal, pretzels, bagels, popcorn, granola, breadsticks, rye wafers, beans, potatoes, sweet potatoes, yams, corn

Protein
Serving Size:
Fist size
1 cup entree
4 ounce meat

(Lean, "select," trim fat are best. Braise, broil, steam, roast, bake, microwave)

Fish, shellfish, eggs (three times per week), beef (chuck steak, round tip, top eye, tenderloin, top sirloin) ,veal, pork (loin/leg, center loin roast, top loin chops, lean ham), wild game, low-fat lunch meat, chicken (white, without skin), turkey (white, without skin)

Dairy
Serving Size:
Thumb size (for cheese),
One cup (for milk, yogurt)

(Low fat, fat free, skim are best)

Milk, yogurt, cheeses (cottage, feta, goat, mozzarella, parmesean, ricotta, skim, American)

Sweets
Serving Size:
One serving size

(Low in fat choices)

Brownie, angel food cake, coffee cake, pudding, cupcake, animal crackers, fruit-filled cookie, gingersnap, graham crackers, wafers, frozen yogurt, soft serve, sherbet, ice milk, sorbet, gelatin, Italian ice

Fats
Serving Size:
One serving size

(Light or fat-free is best; if using regular, not light, then use 1/2 serving size if recipe allows)

Salad dressing, margarine, mayonnaise, nuts*, seeds, vegetable oil, canola oil, olive oil, soybean oil, sunflower oil

*Carbohydrates are complex sugar, so they should be chosen less often so as to control complex sugar intake. Though nuts are high in carbohydrates, certain types are lower in saturated fat, such as hazelnuts, pecans, almonds, and walnuts.

Your Healthzone Plan Tips for Healthy Food Choices

- Enjoy your favorite food, but if you overdo, decrease servings from the carbohydrate category or increase your activities to balance out calories.

- Eat breakfast everyday, as well as a nutritional snack, lunch, another nutritional snack, dinner, and a evening nutritional snack in order to keep your metabolism burning off food and not storing it as fat for future energy. Try to eat six small meals a day.

- If you choose regular salad dressing, butter, ice cream, cheese, etc., keep to one serving size. Consider decreasing carbohydrate intake or increasing exercise to balance calories.

- Choose items that are individually packaged to control serving size.

- Always check the label no matter how small the package is to see how many serving sizes are in the package.

- Enjoy your favorite dessert: try 1/2 the normal serving size and savor it twice as much.

- Large bagels, muffins, slice of bread, etc., may be two serving sizes or more.

- Cereal: most are only 1/2–3/4 cup per serving size.

- Use a salad plate as a dinner plate. Use a coffee cup as a bowl. This can help to keep serving sizes controlled.

- Crave salt or sweet? Crackers and chips or cakes and cookies—you choose; but, keep to one serving size once a day. Decrease carbohydrates and increase exercise for weight maintenance.

- Slow down your eating and savor your food.

- Choose margarine or cooking sprays instead of butter or oils.

- Choosing items that are fresh or frozen increases nutritional levels.

- Choose a vegetable or fruit over fat/salt/sweets.

- Selecting a vegetable or fruit higher in sugar is still better than not selecting a vegetable or fruit at all. Vegetables and fruits provide the bonus of vitamin and mineral nutrition versus the minimal nutrition of a sugary snack.

- For seasoning, try to use herbs and spices instead of syrups, gravies, and sauces.

- Remember: beverages and alcohol calories count.

- Increased carbohydrates=increased complex sugars. So, vegetables and fruits with high carbs may be in the carb category.

- Simple sugar and complex sugar calories not burned off are stored as fat in your body to be used as a future energy source.

- Try to eat breakfast, lunch, and dinner every day to keep your metabolism burning fat and to provide you with constant energy.

- Try nonstick pans and cooking sprays.

- Eat a piece of fruit with breakfast, lunch, and/or while going to/from work or while running errands.

- Cut up vegetables and have them ready and waiting for you in the refrigerator for quick hunger fixes.

- Start dinner with a lettuce salad.

- Make extras of entrees or casseroles to freeze for later. Then microwave for a quick nutritious meal another day.

Eating Out Suggestions

- Choose grilled, broiled, baked, roasted, or poached.

- Ask for butter, syrups, salad dressing, sauces, or gravies on the side.

- Substitute fruit, vegetables, or salad for fries.

- Stop super-sizing to save a few cents; medical care for a heart attack costs more than $20,000, so how much did you really save?

- Use the nutritional information on a label to help you find the healthiest snack. Choose the snack with the most protein, vitamins, minerals, and fiber content, and the least amount of fat and calories per serving.

- Limit alcohol to one 12 ounce beer, or 5 ounce wine, or 1.5 ounce spirits, less than three times a week.

- Enjoy a small nutritious snack and one glass of water before going to a celebration to prevent overeating at the event.

- Look over the buffet food before getting your plate. Use a smaller plate and fill it with a serving size of all your favorites.

- Ask the waiter for a "To Go" container when your meal is served. Immediately put some of your meal into the container to enjoy tomorrow. Refrigerate leftovers properly for your safety.

- Plan ahead for meals and snacks so you're not caught without food plans, that way you won't end up going out to a fast food place.

- Enjoy your favorite foods; savor every morsel in a serving size.

- Overindulged today? Balance it out tomorrow by eating less and exercising more; one single meal, or one single day, can't stop you on your path to better health, exercise, and nutrition.

Healthy Living

Use the Healthzone Plan in this chapter to help you make healthy choices. Follow this plan for 21 days. After 21 days, healthy choices will be a habit that you can follow for life. If you find yourself drifting back to unhealthy habits, pull out the food pyramid and follow the Healthzone Plan again for 21 days. This will get you back into the habit of making healthy choices.

If you feel hungry, first choose items from the vegetable or fruit categories to help you feel full. If you are still hungry, drink a glass of water, eat a small serving of protein, and add more activity or exercise.

Enjoy all foods, savor a serving size. No foods have to be eliminated or forbidden!
Enjoy life in your Healthzone.

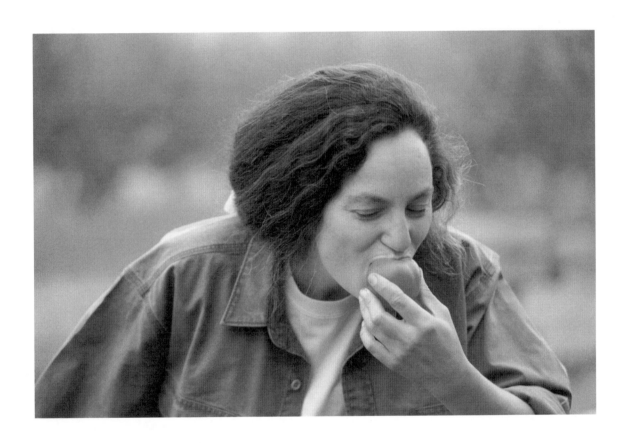

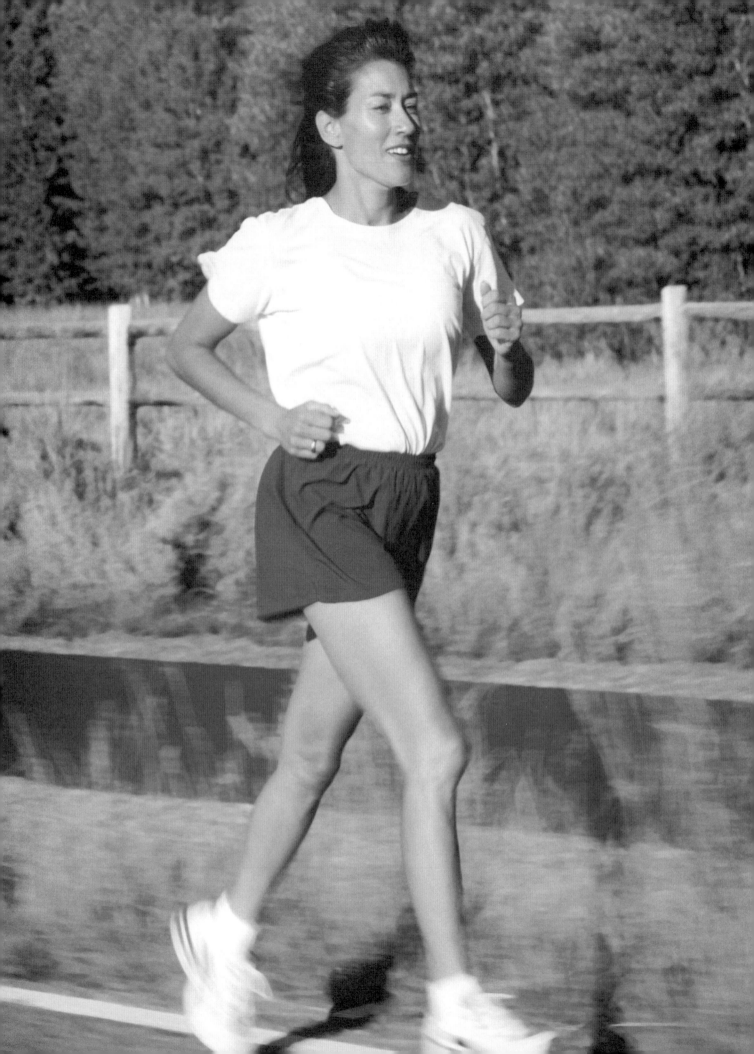

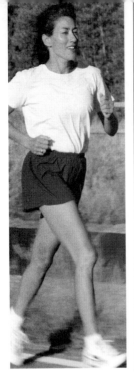

Healthzone

Your lifelong quest to feel good about yourself and to be in harmony, peace and balance with yourself and your environment is completely dependent on you being able to stay within your Healthzone range.

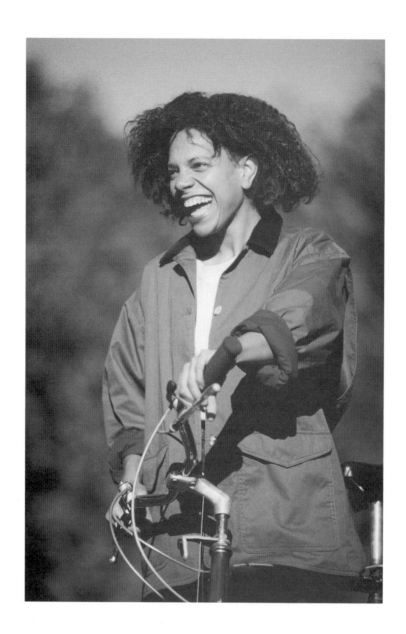

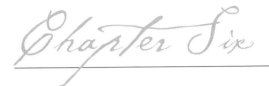

Chapter Six

It is more natural for your body to have a Healthzone range for weight, rather than some exact weight you have assigned to yourself. A weight range allows your body to fluctuate and adjust to your daily life events.

Chapter 6: Redefine Success
Finding Your Personal Healthzone Weight Range

Celebrate, rejoice, and enjoy yourself. You are free. No longer should you define yourself as to whether you are a success or failure by an ideal goal weight that you assigned to yourself when you were 20 years of age. One of the gifts of aging is being able to allow yourself the freedom to redefine who you are, what your image is, and what your goals are. Your life is deeper and richer now than when you were 20; you don't need to define yourself as a good person if you are at your personally assigned ideal weight, or as a bad person if you are not at this personally assigned ideal weight. As a W. Bortz, M.D., article title says, "We Live Too Short and Die Too Long." In other words, we should not spend all of our time making personal sacrifices, denying ourselves, and saying "no" to things in life in order to be an exact weight on a scale.

Your body works in miraculously automatic, rhythmic cycles to keep you functioning and comfortable throughout your day. These rhythmic cycles give your body harmony and balance every moment you live and breathe. Your breathing, heart beat, pulse, sleep cycle, and even the opening and closing of your eyes are all performed automatically by your body's rhythmic cycles without your ever having to give it a second thought. As you go through your day and your body is subjected to changes in your surrounding environment, your body's sensory system is quick to respond and alters your heart rate, pulse, temperature, and breathing to allow you to remain in harmony and balance in your own personal Healthzone. With any challenges it receives throughout your busy day, your body responds automatically to get you back into your Healthzone and range of comfort. When you return to this Healthzone range, you feel harmonious and balanced.

This Healthzone range can apply to all aspects of your life including your spirit, mind, and body. When any element of your spirit, mind, or body drifts out of your personal Healthzone range, you feel disharmony and imbalance. Your lifelong quest to feel good about yourself and be in harmony, peace, and balance with yourself and your environment is completely dependent on your being able to stay within your Healthzone range. If something draws you out of this range, your spirit, mind, and body do everything in their power to help return you to that Healthzone range in order to restore your harmony and balance.

elements of your spirit, mind, or body is drawn away—like a stretching rubber band from this Healthzone core—the core tries to exert a tremendous force on that element and snap it like a rubber band back to your Healthzone core. Think of it this way: your body's weight has a Healthzone range, usually a range of approximately ten pounds around a given weight. If you stay within your ten pound range of this weight, your body rewards you by staying in your Healthzone range and your body's rubber band for weight is at rest and you are, therefore, in harmony and balance in your Healthzone and in your life. Say, however, you have been going to too many parties and are overindulging; you are now stretching your rubber band for your body weight away from your Healthzone. This causes you to feel unhealthy and unbalanced. Stretch your rubber band far enough from your Healthzone range and you see your rubber band for health fragmenting and stretching to a point that the fiber strands start to break and the result is disease— for your body this means "dis-ease." When you stretch your body's rubber band too far from your Healthzone range, you end up with "dis-eases" like heart disease, cancer, and diabetes. Your Healthzone core wants all of your spirit, mind, and body rubber bands back at your Healthzone core to ensure harmony and balance.

When you are able to make lifestyle changes to decrease your body's "dis-ease," your rubber bands stop overstretching, fragmenting, and breaking. When this happens, your sense of well-being is restored. Your body is "healed" or "healthier" and your rubber band fibers are at rest and you are now comfortable. Your sense of well-being is restored because you are in harmony and balance when you stay within your normal range near your Healthzone.

You need to determine your own personal Healthzone range for all aspects of your spirit, mind, and body. When it comes to your body, one body rubber band is your weight. You need to define for yourself what weight range is right for your body's Healthzone range.

In other words, what weight range should you attempt to stay at in order to let your weight rubber bands stay at rest close to your Healthzone? **We all have weight ranges that—if we stay within them— help us feel a better sense of well-being and health. To restrict yourself to one exact weight and say you are only satisfied if you are at that exact weight every moment of every day is unrealistic, unnatural, and sets you up to feel constantly disappointed in yourself.** In addition, this does not allow your body the normal and natural fluctuations it needs to adjust to your constantly changing surrounding environment and life events. Your own heartbeat has a normal and natural Healthzone range from 60–105 beats per minute; it can fluctuate and adjust to the surrounding environment and to your life events. Your weight, too, has a normal and natural Healthzone range that allows you to fluctuate with your surrounding environment and life events.

It is more natural for your body to have a Healthzone range for weight, rather than some exact weight you have assigned yourself. A weight range allows your body to fluctuate and adjust to your daily life events. By allowing yourself the freedom to be creative and flexible with your weight range, you can allow yourself daily variances in your weight but still be in a healthy range for your weight. That way, every day you can celebrate success and feel in control by maintaining your Healthzone for your weight in a range that is right for you.

Healthzone Weight Range

- Determine your healthy weight by looking at the body mass index chart on the next page.*

- Then maintain a Healthzone weight range of 10 pounds around that weight.

- Example: Goal weight=135, so your Healthzone weight range could be from 130–140 pounds.

*Instead of following the body mass index weight chart, you may want to take measurements of your body and follow your success this way. Measurements should include chest, waist, hips, thigh, calf, and upper arm.

Body Mass Index

Height (in feet and inches)

Weight (in pounds)	5'	5'1"	5"2"	5'3"	5'4"	5'5"	5'6"	5'7"	5'8"	5'9"	5'10"	5'11"	6'	6'1"	6'2"
100	20	19	18	18	17	17	16	16	15	15	14	14	14	13	13
105	21	20	19	19	18	17	17	16	16	16	15	15	14	14	13
110	21	21	20	19	19	18	17	17	16	16	16	15	15	15	14
115	22	22	21	20	20	19	19	18	17	17	17	16	16	15	15
120	23	23	22	21	21	20	19	19	18	18	17	17	16	16	15
125	24	24	23	22	21	21	20	20	19	18	18	17	17	16	16
130	25	25	24	23	22	22	21	20	20	19	19	18	18	17	17
135	26	26	25	24	23	22	22	21	21	20	19	19	18	18	17
140	27	26	26	25	24	23	23	22	21	21	20	20	19	18	18
145	28	27	27	26	25	24	23	23	22	21	21	20	20	19	19
150	29	28	27	27	26	25	24	23	23	22	22	21	20	20	19
155	30	29	28	27	27	26	25	24	23	22	22	21	20	20	20
160	31	30	29	28	27	27	26	25	24	24	23	22	22	21	21
165	32	31	30	29	28	27	27	26	25	24	24	23	22	22	21
170	33	32	31	30	29	28	27	27	26	25	24	24	23	22	22
175	34	33	32	31	30	29	28	27	27	26	25	24	24	23	22
180	35	34	33	32	31	30	29	28	27	27	26	25	24	24	23
185	36	35	34	33	32	31	30	29	28	27	27	26	25	24	24
190	37	36	35	34	33	32	31	30	29	28	27	26	26	25	24
195	38	37	36	35	34	33	32	31	30	29	28	27	26	26	25
200	39	38	37	36	35	34	33	32	31	30	29	28	27	26	26
205	40	39	38	37	36	35	34	33	32	31	30	29	28	27	26
210	41	40	38	37	36	35	34	33	32	31	30	29	28	28	27
215	42	41	39	38	37	36	35	34	33	32	31	30	29	28	28
220	43	42	40	39	38	37	36	35	34	33	32	31	30	29	28
225	44	43	41	40	39	37	36	35	34	33	32	31	31	30	29
230	45	43	42	41	39	38	37	36	35	34	33	32	31	30	30
235	46	44	43	42	40	39	38	37	36	35	34	33	32	31	30

☐ **Less than 19: Underweight—at underweight health risk**

☐ **19–26: Satisfactory—normal healthy weight-to-height ratio**

◼ **27–30: Overweight—at increased health risk**

◼ **Greater than 30: Obese—at considerable health risk**

BMI Chart Courtesy of Dr. Raymond Cole, from his book Osteoporosis: Unmasking a Silent Thief © 2000 Dr. Raymond Cole and Wellmark Publications

Redefine Success: Maintaining Your Healthzone Weight Range Health Tips

- Today, remember that your goal is better health and enhanced well-being. By being near your Healthzone, you restore harmony and balance to your spirit, mind, and body.

- Prepare for your success. Celebrate by rewarding yourself with a treat (i.e. a new CD, outfit, or a flower for your garden).

- Choose a weight range and stay 10 pounds around this weight. Believe in yourself to achieve. Choose one serving size for food and make time to do daily activities to maintain your weight.

- **Design a plan for increased activity that works for you. Schedule the time in your daily planner. Walking is excellent. Increased activity keeps you happier, healthier, mentally sharp, toned, and feeling better. Increase your activities and you get to eat more. Want a chocolate malt? That's 350 calories, which equals 30 minutes on the treadmill. So, after 30 minutes on the treadmill, all of the calories from the chocolate malt are burned off.**

- Increasing your daily activities helps keep you in your Healthzone weight range. You can accumulate your five to ten minutes of activities by taking the stairs at work, parking further from the building and walking, standing while talking on the phone, weeding your garden, or sweeping the kitchen floor to total 30 minutes of exercise daily and have near equal benefits when compared to a 30-minute aerobic workout.

- **Be creative, be flexible, and have several choices when selecting foods and activities. The beauty of the Healthzone is that it allows you to be you. Just choose within your range of comfort and you can enjoy yourself at any event. Baseball game: have the hot dog and enjoy it, eat less for dinner, or walk that day.**

- Enjoy a variety of foods and eat three to six small meals daily. Eat slowly and savor your food. Use the good silverware and cloth napkins to create a pleasant dining experience.

- Enjoy five fruits and vegetables daily. The crunching is very satisfying to your soul. Drink 64 ounces of water daily. Eat 25 grams of fiber daily.

- **Discover a new routine to get rid of your old, unhealthy eating habits. To look different than you do now, you are going to have to do something differently. Sit in a different TV chair, try a healthier snack. Changing your habits will reward you with success.**

- Break the night fast with a good breakfast. It is a must to jump-start your metabolism to help your body burn calories more efficiently all day long.

- Indulge in the comforts of stimulating your senses with art, music, and hobbies instead of the comforts of food.

- Savor your life instead of savoring food. Savor a sunset, a movie, or a call to a friend.

- Make one healthier food choice today. Eating healthier helps regulate your blood sugar, decrease heart disease, control your appetite and cravings, increase your energy, decrease stress, and increase your sense of well-being.

- Being in your Healthzone tastes great. No food tastes as good as being in your Healthzone feels.

- Enjoy all foods a cup or less at a time. Pre-plan meals and snacks. Make another choice if you crave more than a cup full (or fist full) proportion size of any food. Consider filling up, instead, with fresh air, sunshine, or with a walk.

- **Enjoy yourself, feel good, and have fun in life while being in your health range for your Healthzone.**

- Your #1 investment should be you. Choose to be healthy, so you will be around to enjoy all those stocks and bonds, savings, 401K, and retirement funds that you have been working so hard to have in your future.

**Congratulate yourself. Give yourself the permission to like and care about yourself.
Allow yourself to be a success at being the best you can be.**

Yes It Does Count! Even if...

- It is a quick lick while no one is watching.

- You don't sit down to eat it.

- It is fat free or low calorie.

- No one sees you sneak a bite.

- It is liquid.

- It does not taste good.

- You take a taste of someone else's food.

- You take a taste while cooking.

- You are eating while watching TV or driving, and don't remember eating.

- And just to keep things interesting, did you know that sugar has no fat and vegetable oil has no cholesterol?

Be the BEST you can be by believing in yourself to achieve success in your customized Healthzone.

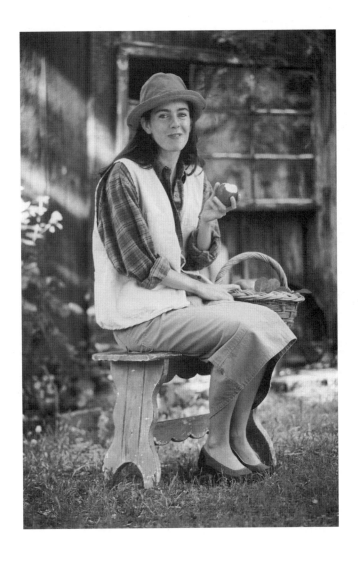

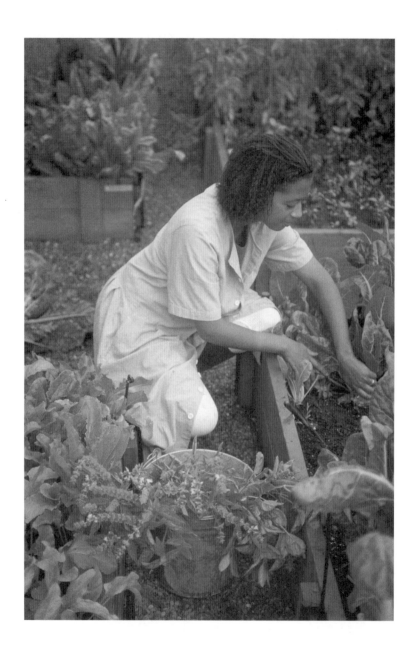

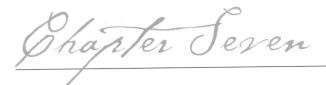

Chapter Seven

Instead of looking weak and helpless, withering away in a long-term care facility, some people may have been able to remain strong and free—living independently and enjoying a robust, fulfilling life shared with others.

Chapter 7: Be Strong
Discover Your Inner Power

It was my third year of medical residency and each one of us in my residency class had been assigned to care for patients in a nursing home while doing our other medical training duties. The goal was to provide us "new doctors" with the medical knowledge in the field of geriatrics (medicine for patients over 65 years old). It was also supposed to give us an insight into the aging process in the human body and how aging affects the geriatrician's overall well-being.

I remember this particular day as being an absolutely gorgeous fall day as I made my way from the nursing home parking lot towards the nursing home front door; I lingered in the parking lot, brushing my foot through the spectrum of orange, red, and yellow leaves underneath my feet, enjoying the crunching sound as I pressed my foot down onto the leaves. I raised my eyes to the blue sky speckled with puffs of white clouds, and inhaled the fresh, crisp fall air. Soaking in the last seconds of this wonderful fall moment, I entered the nursing home front door and was greeted by a blast of heat that instantly flushed my cheeks. The room temperature had to have been over 80 degrees; it was very uncomfortable. Yet, the nursing home residents sitting in the entry lounge had on sweaters and lap blankets. My nostrils were overwhelmed by the pungent nursing home odors that greeted me. As I made my way past the information desk and towards the nursing station, I simply could not get past the overpowering odor of stool in the air. The odor seemed to follow me down the hallway.

In front of me, two nurses were pushing a resident in a geriatric shower chair (looks like a toilet seat on wheels with steel arms and back rest) used for patients who are unable to bathe or shower themselves. A patient sits nude on this "throne" while being showered by the nurses. I slowed my pace near the nurse's station as the two nurses pushed the resident in the geriatric shower chair through the doorway into the shower room. I looked to see what had dropped from the patient as the patient was being pushed through the doorway. I couldn't believe my eyes—it was stool. The patient being pushed to the shower in the geriatric shower chair had expelled stool (involuntarily) all the way down the hallway.

In horror, my eyes followed the fresh stool trail all the way down the hallway that had dropped from the patient in the geriatric shower chair all the way from the patient's room to the shower room. No wonder it smelled so bad in the hallway. Immediately, I checked my shoes. Fortunately, no surprises.

At the nurse's station there were more residents lined in up geriatric chairs (straight-backed wooden chairs on wheels). Most were seat belted into these chairs. There was an attached tray to the arm rest for food and drink. Some residents were very alert and social, appearing to have a good mind, but their body was being held prisoner in an aging, disabled body. Others were in various stages of alertness. Most of the residents I had seen up to this point could not have provided for themselves in any basic way such as bathing, teeth brushing, or hair maintenance. The residents I saw that morning were not able to drive a car or clean an apartment—let alone prepare a meal for themselves. If put to the test, most probably would not even have been able to lift a gallon of milk (less than 10 pounds).

If you could push a button to rewind time to when the nursing home residents were in their 40s and 50s, their lives could probably have played out very differently, if only they had done a small amount of daily exercise to invest for a future of independence and freedom. Instead of looking weak and helpless, withering away in a long term care facility, some may have been able to remain strong and free and living independently enjoying a robust, fulfilling life shared with others in their golden years.

You say your life is too busy right now to devote any time to yourself for exercise or weight lifting? STOP! Rewind now and reverse those thoughts. You don't have the time NOT to start exercising right now. Right now, wherever you are in your life is the right time to start exercising. **Whether you are working, or a stay-at-home-Mom—whatever your individual scenario—every movement of exercise you make now is an investment in your future health, strength, independence, and freedom.** Never been an exerciser? It's not you? Never lifted a weight in your lifetime? No bulky look for you? Rethink it! Even lifting a gallon of milk is a form of weight lifting. If it makes you feel unfeminine to lift weights, get over it! Grab a 16-ounce can of chili in each hand and use that for your toning. **This is not about bulking up, rippling muscles, or preparing to enter body building competitions. This is about doing a little stretching, toning, and firming investment for your muscles now so that you can be strong, independent, and free in order to enjoy yourself your entire life and not be bound to a geriatric chair.**

If you think you don't have time to exercise, I challenge you to keep a diary for two days. You will be surprised to see your newspaper, magazine, novel, TV, news, etc., time add up. Squeeze out 30 to 45 minutes a day. If you spend 30 minutes a day reading a paper, then you can spend 30 minutes a day exercising. Can't give up the newspaper? Then get a reading rack and put it in front of you on a bike, treadmill, etc. Still can't find the time? Get up 30 minutes earlier; you will enjoy the peace and quiet of the world and be treated to a spectacular sunrise to start your day with a smile on your face, and the knowledge that you got a jump-start on better health before you were even fully awake.

Exercise and weight lifting allows you to have more energy than you have had in years. It helps to slow down the aging process. It strengthens your muscles. It decreases body fat. It decreases injury due to weakness (you can't open a fire door because it knocks you over, lifting a one-gallon milk jug is too heavy for you—so you drop it and break your osteoporotic foot).

Exercise and lifting weights also allows you to have solid bones, increases your metabolism to allow you to burn off that cheesecake you ate earlier, and increases your flexibility to reach those bike pedals and stretch for the handlebars. Weight lifting allows you to lose weight by burning more calories every day and increases your endurance to get from one end of the outlet mall to the other in record time (without even having to drive your car to the stores located at the other end of the mall).

Your muscles are your friends and they want to be moved. They are the happiest and serve you the best when they are given a little motion. **It doesn't matter to your muscles what age you are or what your previous level of conditioning has been.** With just a little bit of investment of time now, whether it be gardening, or exercise machines a few times a week, your muscles will be able to spring into action at a moment's notice to get you into any activity your heart desires.

Don't let your mind be trapped in an aging, disabled body. Broaden your horizons and vision and let your imagination open up to take you to a fitness level you have never achieved before. Your muscles do not show significant signs of aging unless you don't use them. If you don't use them, they shrink down and are only of a minimum benefit to you and can only give you a minimum amount of support for daily activities. All it takes is a few repetitions using 1–10 pound weights a few times a week. That is it!

Weight lifting using 1–10 pound weights a few times a week is your ticket to future freedom and independence. **You will lose weight, tone up, trim down, firm up, strengthen your bones, have more flexibility, decrease body fat, gain energy, and burn calories (even while at rest) because of your increased metabolism.** You will feel empowered and in control of your body. You will be more fit. Your muscles will enable you to keep up with your significant other on a bike ride, go on a walk with a friend, or join your kids playing tennis.

Allow yourself the chance to be able to engage in any activity you desire. Shatter your own personal records. Set your bar higher. Stop limiting your activities by mentally sabotaging yourself. You can do it. Your body will respond quickly to your efforts. What are you waiting for? Your body and muscles are raring to go. With just a tiny amount of effort on your part and low pound weights, your body will respond quickly and snap itself into a new shape. Your body wants you to feel good and be fit. You will be totally amazed at discovering how strong and fit and free you can feel if you just give yourself 21 days to try these moves a few times a week for the next few weeks. You will be totally amazed by how quickly your body's muscles respond to a minimal effort, and you will be amazed at the fast results. **Get up and get off the sidelines and get on the playing field of life. Be empowered, free, and in control. Discover the power that is inside of you, waiting for you to get started.**

Feel Great
Feel your power. Be free. Be strong.

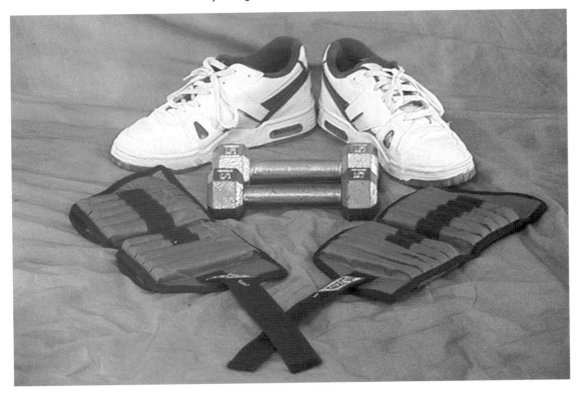

Photo courtesy of Dr. Raymond Cole from Best Body, Best Bones © 2001 Dr. Raymond Cole and Wellmark Publications

A simple investment for your success.

Your Secret to Feeling Great

Walking
30 Minutes, Monday through Saturday

Toning
Upper Body: 15–30 Minutes, Monday, Wednesday, and Friday
(using 1–10 pound hand weights)
Lower Body: 15–30 Minutes, Tuesday, Thursday, and Saturday
(using 1–2 pound ankle weights)
Sunday: Free day! Enjoy your favorite activity!

This is all you need to get started creating a new you!*

Upper Body Exercises
Monday, Wednesday, Friday, do 12 repetitions of each exercise, working your way up to 3 sets of 12 repetitions.

Exercise 1

Step 1

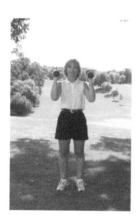

Starting position

Step 2

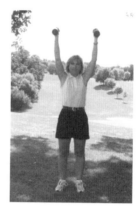

Reach hands straight up.

Exercise 2

Step 1

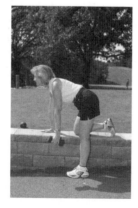

Starting position

Step 2

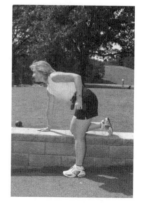

Bend elbow and draw back and up.
Complete set, then repeat using other arm.

*Consult your doctor before starting any exercise program.

Upper Body Exercises continued

Exercise 3

Step 1
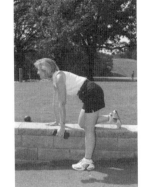
Starting position

Step 2
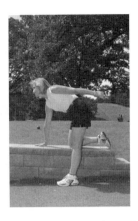
Draw straight arm back and up.
Complete set, then repeat using other arm.

Exercise 4

Step 1
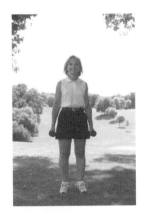
Starting position

Step 2
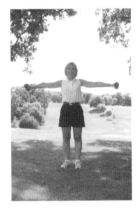
Lift arms up and out to shoulder height.

Exercise 5

Step 1
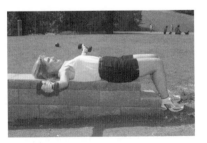
Starting position

Step 2
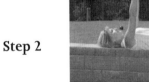
Bring straight arms upward and
bring hands together.

Exercise 6

Step 1
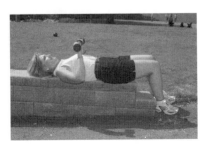
Starting position

Step 2
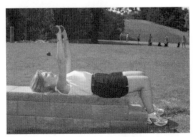
Push hands upward, straightening arms.

Upper Body Exercises continued

Exercise 7

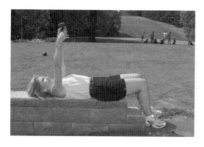

Step 1

Starting position

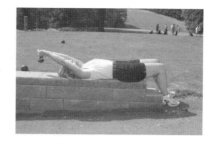

Step 2

Draw straight arms back, above head.

Exercise 8

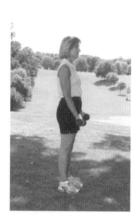

Step 1

Starting position

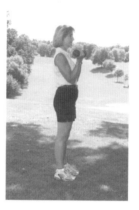

Step 2

Bend elbows, raising weights to chest.

Lower Body Exercises

Tuesday, Thursday, Saturday, do 12 repetitions of each exercise, working your way up to 3 sets of 12 repetitions.

Exercise 1

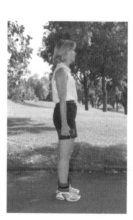

Step 1

Starting position

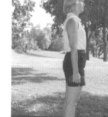

Step 2

Lift heels off ground and hold briefly.

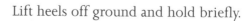

Lower Body Exercises continued

Exercise 2

Step 1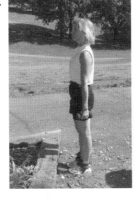

Starting position

Step 2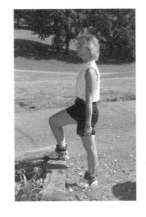

Raise right foot onto step

Step 3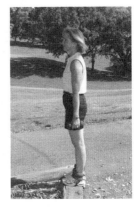

Raise left foot onto step. Return right foot, then left foot, to ground. Repeat steps, using left foot first.

Exercise 3

Step 1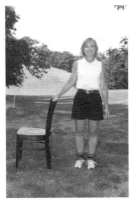

Starting position

Step 2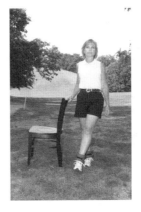

Raise foot and cross straight leg over balanced leg. Complete set, then repeat with other leg

Exercise 4

Step 1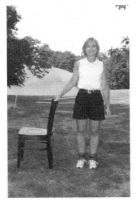

Starting position

Step 2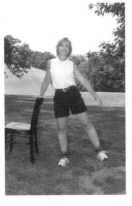

Raise straight arm and leg to side. Complete set, then repeat on other side

Lower Body Exercises continued

Exercise 5

Step 1

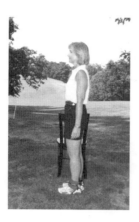

Starting position

Step 2

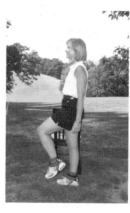

Bend and lift knee. Complete set,
then repeat with opposite leg.

Exercise 6

Step 1

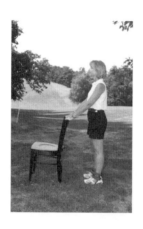

Starting position

Step 2

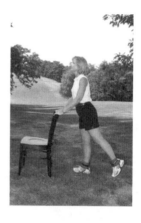

Raise foot, keeping leg straight.
Complete set, then repeat with other leg.

Exercise 7

Step 1

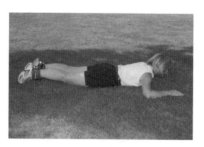

Starting position

Step 2

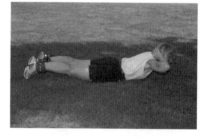

Lift head and feet off of ground,
arching upward.

Exercise 8

Step 1

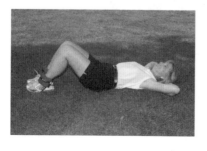

Starting position

Step 2

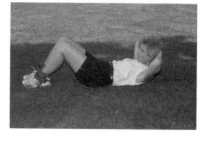

Lift head, arms, and upper torso up and
forward, toward legs.

What if I were to tell you that FOR FREE you could have:

- More energy
- More strength
- Better sleep
- Better sex
- Improved self esteem
- Improved brain power
- Lowered risk of disease (high blood pressure, stroke, heart disease, cancer of breast or colon, diabetes)
- More happiness
- More endorphins (natural feel good chemicals)
- More agility
- More freedom to say "yes" to impulse athletic activities (without having to take the time to get in shape)
- A feeling of being fit and fabulous!

These benefits are all yours FOR FREE! All you have to do is start your body moving. You can own every one of these benefits through exercise. You don't have to push yourself to the brink of exhaustion to get these benefits. These benefits are free, even with the smallest effort of exercise. Just be consistent to get the results. It is never too late to get started, no matter what your age or previous lifestyle. Your body's better health will reward your effort. All your body wants in order to be happy and good to you is a little movement—you will be amazed at the results in just 21 days. So, let your mind help your body unleash its power.

Here is a plan that is perfect for you:

- 30 minutes walking (or any aerobic activity) daily
- 15 minutes toning and firming with light weights, alternate days for upper and lower body
- One free day to enjoy your favorite activity

That is it! It is as easy and simple as that to be healthier, happier, more fit, and have the strength to indulge in life to the fullest. You will have the freedom to partake in spur-of-the-moment activities like playing tennis, taking a bike ride, planting your garden, etc. Say "yes" to your health, and to being fit and fabulous. Take the time right now to exercise for a happier, healthier future. Invest in yourself for a few minutes daily, and receive—for free—a more enhanced quality of life. You're worth it!

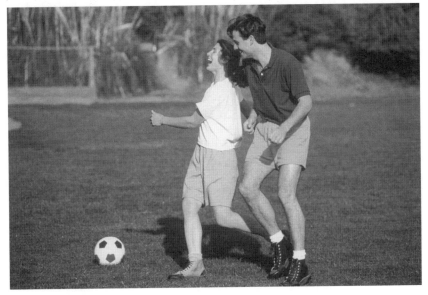

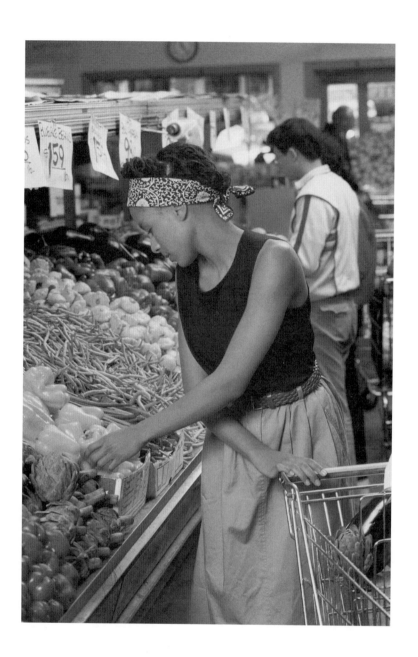

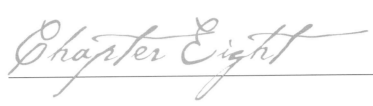

Chapter Eight

Watch out for marketing ploys and claims that will leave your pocketbook drained and your shelves bursting with bottles of hope that promise better nutrition and health. If the products you see being advertised make promises that seem too good to be true—they probably are.

Chapter 8: Vitamins, Minerals, and Herbs

If you eat a sensible and balanced diet you do not need to take a vitamin or supplement, right? Are the handfuls of vitamins and supplements you see friends putting into their bodies really healthy for them?

In our society of quick, convenient, and processed foods is there any more nutrition in the food that we eat than in the box that it came from? After your food has been picked, processed, heated, chilled, stored, and reheated, there may not be much nutrition remaining.

In an attempt to provide more nutrition in food, supplementation can be added to certain foods. For instance, folate has been added to flour and cereal products to help women who are trying to conceive to decrease neural tube defects in their baby. Milk is fortified with vitamin D which helps you absorb calcium easier. Calcium helps to decrease bone loss, and prevent osteopenia and osteoporosis, thus decreasing your chances of getting a fracture.

The very best way to get your vitamins and minerals is to eat at least five servings of a variety of fresh fruits and vegetables a day. If you are able to grow your own fruits and vegetables, all the better! The fresher and less processed your food, the more nutritious. Farmers markets, organically grown, fresh produce aisles, and fresh frozen products all provide good sources for nutrition. The more processed: chopped, diced, cooked, canned, or boxed items are, the less nutrition they have.

When you eat natural and fresh fruits and vegetables you are provided with hundreds of natural antioxidants, flavonoids, and carotenoids. These are thought to help prevent certain diseases such as heart disease and cancer.

If you find that you are getting your nutrition by mainly eating your way though fast food restaurants, and boxes and cans of processed foods, you are probably getting **suboptimal levels** of vitamins and minerals. **You could benefit from taking one multivitamin a day**. Always remember to tell your doctor what vitamins, minerals, or herbs that you are taking. These can sometimes affect your other medicines or cause a drug side effect.

You should choose a multivitamin that has the currently recommended amount of vitamins and minerals. The term, recommended daily allowance (RDA), is being replaced by the new term, reference daily intakes (RDI). The RDI is the new recommended daily values of vitamins and minerals you should take.

For most people, taking large amounts of additional supplements of vitamins and minerals is not necessary and may actually be harmful or toxic, so beware! The vitamin and mineral industry is not currently regulated by the Food and Drug Administration (FDA). **Watch out for marketing ploys and claims that will leave your pocketbook drained and your shelves bursting with bottles of hope that promise better nutrition and health.** If the products you see being advertised make promises that seem too good to be true—they probably are.

Sound advice that has stood the test of time remains; do what your mother told you to do—eat your fruits and vegetables.

Vitamins: A Closer Look

Eating a sensible and balanced diet complete with five servings of fruits and vegetables, and taking just one multivitamin a day should provide 100 percent of the recommended reference daily intake (RDI) of most vitamins and minerals. Unless your doctor has advised you to take extra supplementation, avoid taking more than 100 percent of any vitamin or mineral.

Please use the chart on the following page as your reference guide to the listed vitamins and minerals.

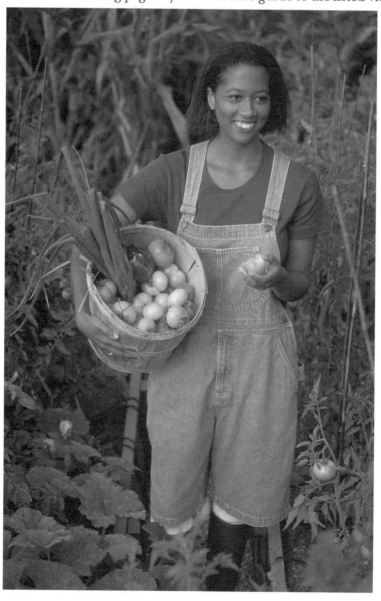

Vitamins	Daily value*	Natural Sources	Benefits	Deficiency Symptoms	Toxicity Symptoms
Vitamin A (fat soluble)***	5000 IU	animal product, beta-carotene, green, yellow, or orange fruits	antioxidant**, better vision, improves immunity, skin repair	night blindness, increased infections, dry hair or skin	liver toxicity, vision changes, increased hip fracture, cracks in lips, yellow skin, hair loss, peeling skin
Vitamin C (water soluble)	60 mg	citrus fruits, strawberries, melons, tomatoes, peppers, broccoli	antioxidant, make collagen for strong skin, heals wounds, makes hormones, helps absorbs iron	bruising, easy bleeding, poor wound healing, soft gums, weakness, pinpoint broken blood vessels under skin	diarrhea, nausea, increased calcium oxalate stones formed, stomach upset
Vitamin E (fat soluble)	30 IU	salad oils, nuts, margarine, beans, veggies, veg. oil, seeds	antioxidant, improves immunity, repairs tissue, decreases leg cramps, decreases premenstrual syndrome	weakness, imbalance, irregular menstrual	stomach upset, bleeding, fatigue, cramps, diarrhea
Vitamin D (fat soluble)	400 IU	body makes w/ sunlight exposure, milk, salt water fish, egg	helps body absorb calcium, decreases bone fractures, strong teeth	bone loss, osteopenia, osteoporosis, fractures, rickets****, burning mouth, insomnia, decreased appetite	extra calcium in tissue and blood, weakness
Vitamin K (fat soluble)	60 mcg	body makes with intestine bacteria, dark green veg., egg yoke, oats, wheat	helps normal blood clotting, helps build bone	increased bleeding, prolonged antibiotic use can lower vit K production in intestines increasing diarrhea	flushing, sweating
Vitamin B12 (water soluble)	6 mcg	animal products, meat, fish, egg, milk	helps make protein and blood, helps burn fat and carbs, higher energy, lower stress, protects nerve endings	anemia (pernicious), numbness, fatigue, memory loss, moodiness, ringing in ears	

*If you have special dietary needs, you may need different daily values than listed.

**Antioxidants decrease cancer, inhibit aging, and bind free radicals in order to prevent disease.

***Fat soluble can become toxic more easily than water soluble (you get rid of water soluble more easily).

****Rickets results in weak bones and profuse sweating.

© 2002 Dr. Robin Hartley

Vitamin chart continued on following page

Vitamins	Daily Value*	Natural Sources	Benefits	Deficiency Symptoms	Toxicity Symptoms
Folate (folic acid) (water soluble)	400 mcg (.4 mg) (800 mg if trying to get pregnant)	dark, leafy veg. whole grain cereals, grains, flour, dairy, animal products	decreases homocysteine** levels, decreases neural tube defects in a fetus, increased energy	anemia, red or sore tongue, fatigue, insomnia, weakness	
Coenzyme Q10		salmon, beef mackerel, peanuts, spinach	antioxidant, increased energy, increased immunity, increased tissue oxygen, decreased allergy symptoms	increased blood sugar, gum disease	
B1 (thiamine)	1.5 mg	egg yolks, fish, beans, grains	antioxidant, helps form blood, burns carbs, increases brain function	Beriberi,*** constipation, fatigue, forgetfulness, numbness, tingling, weak muscles	
B2 (riboflavin)	1.7 mg	cheese, egg yolks, fish, beans, meat, milk, grains, yogurt	makes red blood cells, increases oxygen used by tissues, decreased carpal tunnel	cracks and sores in mouth corners, swollen tongue, dizziness, hair loss	
B3 (niacin)	20 mg	liver, broccoli, carrots, cheese, eggs, fish, milk	improved skin and nerves, lowers cholesterol	Pellagra,**** canker sores, depression, diarrhea, fatigue headache	marked flushing, rash
B5 (pantothenic acid)	10 mg	beef, yeast, eggs, veggies, beans	decreases stress, helps make hormones and antibodies, increases energy	fatigue, stomach upset, burning feet	
B6 (pyridoxine)	2.0 mg	eggs, fish, meat, wheat germ, spinach, carrots, potatoes	helps physical and mental health, decreases homocysteine	anemia, seizures, nausea, sore tongue, headaches	hand and feet numbness and tingling, headache

*If you have special dietary needs, you may need different daily values than listed.

**Increased homocysteine levels can cause increased risk of heart disease.

***BeriBeri symptoms include weakness, tingling, numbness.

****Pellagra symptoms include red, itchy skin and stomach upset.

Minerals	Daily* Value	Natural Sources	Benefits	Deficiency Symptoms	Toxicity Symptoms
Calcium (body will only absorb 500 mg at a time so spread out intake)	1,000–1,200 mg (1,500 mg if postmenopausal) need to take with vitamin D	dairy, green leafy veg., sardine, salmon, broccoli, oats, cabbage, seeds	strong teeth, bones, muscle strength, decreased muscle cramps	achy joints, brittle nails, eczema, insomnia, numbness in legs and arms, fractures	increased kidney stones, interferes iron and zinc absorption, severe constipation
Magnesium	400 mg	meat, fish, dairy, seafood, fruits, vegetables	regulates heart beat, helps lower fatigue of muscle or nerves, helps PMS, helps absorb calcium	rapid heartbeat, weakness, irritability, insomnia	irregular heartbeat, decreased blood pressure, shortness of breath
Iron	18 mg	green leafy veg. meat, liver, whole cereal, grains	increased energy, increased blood and muscle cells, increased immunity	anemia, brittle hair, fatigue, pale skin color, hair loss, groves in fingernails	
Selenium	55 mcg	grains, meats, dairy, chicken, vegetables, whole grains	antioxidant, improves immunity, increases alertness, increases antibodies	fatigue, increased infections	joint aches, brittle nails, stomach upset, hair loss, irritability, metal taste in mouth
Potassium		dairy, fruit, veg., fish, meat, whole grains	regulates heartbeat, pancreas needs to make insulin, helps muscles contract	dry skin, chills, depression, swelling, irregular heartbeat, abnormal blood pressure, weakness	irregular heartbeat
Omega-3		herring, nuts, sardines, salmon, mackerel, seeds, fish oil, beans, soy bean oil, veg. oil	decrease cholesterol and triglycerides, decrease blood clots, helps make prostaglandins, heart beneficial		
Omega-6		deepwater fish, fish and canola oil	same as Omega-3 above		
Glucosamine (amino sugar)	500 mg (3 times a day)	body makes, supplements	helps make bone, tendon ligament, nails, helps arthritis and bursitis		

*If you have special dietary needs, you may need different daily values than listed.

© 2002 Dr. Robin Hartley

Herbs: A Closer Look

Currently, herbal medicine is a 13 billion dollar industry. Herbal remedies have been used for a long time in other countries. In some European countries, herbs are regulated by the government; in these countries, they have to be proven safe, have efficacy, and be of consistent quality in order to be sold.

In the United States, vitamins, minerals, and herbs are unregulated. To date, there are no government guidelines for manufacturers to follow. It is expected that guidelines will be forthcoming in the future; but until standards are set, the manufacturers are expected to follow the food industry's "good manufacturing practices." A product must be unsafe before the FDA will step in and restrict its usage.

You should tell your doctor about any vitamins, minerals, or herbs you are taking. If you do decide to take one of these products, discuss it with your doctor to avoid a toxicity or drug interaction.

Please use the chart on the following page as your reference guide to the listed herbs.

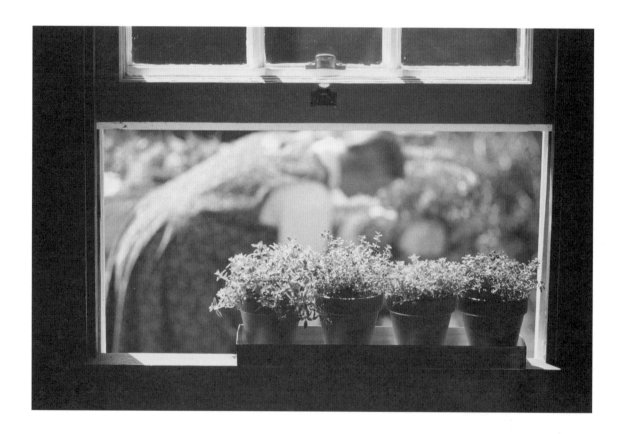

Herb	Part Used	Claims (action)	Risks	Drug Interactions
St. John's wort (Hypericum perforatum)	flowers, leaves, stem	decreases mild depression, increases sedation	flushing, rashes, GI upset, constipation, sun sensitivity	with coumadin, birth control, Digoxin, iron, and antidepressant
Ginkgo biloba (Ginkgo biloba)	leaves, seeds	antioxidant, increased circulation, increased memory, decreased anxiety	increased bleeding, GI upset, rash, cramps	
Ginseng (Panax ginseng)	roots	increased energy, lowered stress, increased appetite, increase athletic ability	high blood pressure, vaginal bleeding, increased sleepiness, increased edema	with coumadin. Don't use if you have high blood pressure, heart disease, or low blood sugar.
Echinacea (Echinacea pallida)	leaves, roots	increased immunity, decreased inflammation	do not take for longer than a few days	
Saw palmetto (Serenoa repens)	berries, seeds, fruits	increased urination, increased appetite	GI upset	
Kava Kava (Piper methysticum)	roots	increased relaxation, improved sleep, increased urination	rash	alprazolam, causes drowsiness
Ephedra (Ephedra sinica) (Ma-Huang)	stems, roots	stimulant, decongestant, increased mood, decreased appetite	high blood pressure , heart palpitations, seizure, stroke, kidney stones, moodiness, rapid heartbeat, vomiting, sleepiness, nausea	don't use if you have anxiety, heart disease, high blood pressure, or glaucoma
Black cohosh (Cimicifuga racemosa)	roots	decreased hot flashes, decreased cramps	vomit, headache, dizzy, decreased blood pressure, limb pain, GI upset, limit to 6 mo.	don't use if you have a chronic disease
Evening Primrose oil (Oenothera biennis)	seeds	decreased PMS, hot flashes, and menopause symptoms, flaking of skin and itching		
Red clover (Trifolium pratense)	flowers	decreased menopause symptoms, cough suppressant	appetite suppressed	

Tips for Vitamins, Minerals, and Herbs:

- Do not self-medicate! Get an accurate diagnosis for your symptoms from your doctor before taking any product.
- More is not better. Take only the recommended dose (if okayed by your doctor).
- Natural products can still have serious side effects.
- Select from respected manufacturers to avoid product substitution or altered products.
- A good reference source is http://ods.od.nih.gov/databases/ibids.html, provided by the office of dietary supplements at the National Institutes of Health.
- Start with a low dosage and go slowly up to the recommended doses to avoid side effects (if okayed by your doctor).

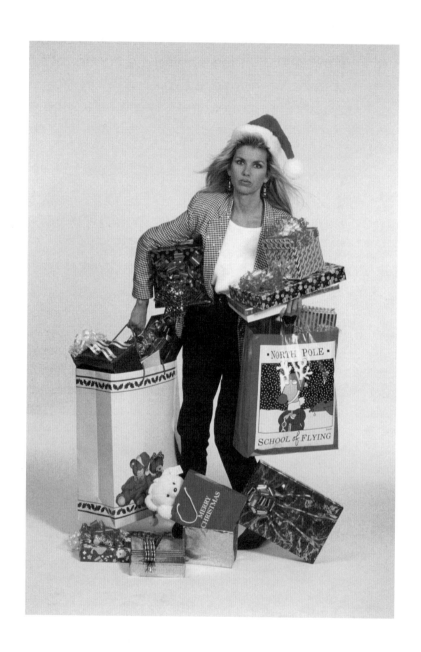

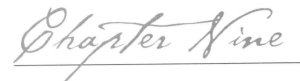

Chapter Nine

Introduction of new milestones such as parenting your parents or understanding the hormonal surges of your newly "teenaged" children can conflict with your raging hormones; this can be challenging, emotionally draining, and exhausting.

Chapter 9: Not Tonight Dear, I Have... Way Too Much To Do

Not tonight dear, I have way too much to do, and I am way too tired from all that had to be done today to make any time for you now! Earlier in the week it had sounded so good to promise Saturday night to your partner. You were certain that you would be reenergized and ready for action on an emotional, mental, and physical level by Saturday. You even made suggestive promises throughout the week about the adventures that lie ahead for Saturday night. Finally, Saturday arrives, and it started out with its usual "bang!"

Bolting out of bed at the crack of dawn, you spend the day racing through your children's activities: basketball games, soccer practices and games, math tutoring class, and the end of the soccer season pizza luncheon (weren't you supposed to buy the coach's "thank you" gift?).

You charge back home after the last afternoon soccer game to start preparing dinner for your family—and the 17 guests you invited over earlier in the week when you were feeling guilty because you and your partner never see any of your friends anymore. You were feeling optimistic that it would be fun to have everyone over. Your guests arrive, and you try to look like the calm "hostess with the mostess" as you wait for your partner to get home from your other son's soccer tournament. You shed a tear (of joy?) when your son's team didn't advance to the finals, and your partner has finally arrived home to help with the dinner party.

It is now 11:30 p.m. and the last of the guests have left, the kitchen is semi-clean, the dishwasher crammed full of things that are *supposed to be* dishwasher safe, and the handwash-only items are all that remain cluttering the counter to greet you in the morning. You drag yourself up the stairs to the bedroom to make a halfhearted attempt to do your nightly "beauty" ritual (face cream that promises an eyelift from a jar), brush your teeth with a whitener, and swap your flattering hostess outfit for your comfy, tattered flannel PJ's. All the while, you avoid looking at your body in the mirror while you are changing—who needs that reminder before bedtime that you *really* need to start doing toning exercises?

Finally, you flop into bed—and then you notice your patiently waiting, apprehensive partner in bed who reminds you of your suggestive promises that you had made earlier in the week. You *are* in the mood, aren't you? Of course *he* is in the mood, *he* has taken a Viagra pill.

Your sexual attitudes and desires have been evolving and forming over your entire lifetime. Who you have become and who you are today represents years of a personal journey that has taken you down many paths. Your attitude towards sex and your attitude towards your body have been formed by your experiences, emotions, and values. This includes your feelings of what "good girls" do, your history of abuse, guilt, fear of intimacy, religious values, and concerns about pregnancy. These all shape your attitude about sex and your body image.

What is "normal" according to others may not be normal for you. When you better understand your sexual beliefs and values, you can come closer to being your personal best by the standards that you customize to fit your own needs. When you set the sexual standards that are right for you, then you are able to have a better overall level of sexual satisfaction. As you approach your 40s and beyond, there are many life events that compete for your time and attention. At one point in your life, you may have felt that sex equals babies, and now that your reproductive role is completed, so is your sexual functioning.

Introduction to new milestones—such as parenting your parents or understanding the hormonal surges of your "newly teenaged" children—can conflict with your raging, changing hormones. This can be challenging, emotionally draining, and exhausting. Life events such as a job loss, career changes or retirement, death of a loved one, or a child spreading her/his wings and flying away (soaring as you have taught her/him to do), all pull at your heart strings and leave little time left over for you and your spouse. Add to all of this your changing body, and it can cause you to feel less than desirable.

As you age, your body is going through many changes. Your hormone levels are changing— causing hot flashes, sleep disturbances, night sweats, and possibly a decline in sexual desire. You may have an irregular menses cycle surging and purging unpredictably. Your vaginal mucosa is thinning and is drier. Decreased blood flow, a tightened vaginal opening, decreased elasticity, itching, and burning can all make for painful or unpleasant intercourse. You may be experiencing urinary incontinence that can make intercourse embarrassing. You may be taking a medication, such as an antidepressant, that takes away your sex drive. A tilted uterus, bladder, rectum, or even surgical scars may make intercourse uncomfortable. Or you may have a medical reason for your decreased sexual function such as a thyroid disorder, heart disease, diabetes, or endometriosis. With all this, no wonder you may not be in the mood. **Intercourse should not be painful, physically or mentally—if it is, see your doctor.**

One of my friends, while desperately trying to get pregnant before "her clock ran out of time," briefly saw intercourse as just a way to get pregnant. She would only take off one pant leg for her husband to do his mission. When the mission was accomplished, she would put her pant leg back on and return to whatever she was previously doing. Now that is being focused.

Another woman said she gives her husband a two day window of opportunity each month to have intercourse with her. She is hands off—don't even think about it—during the PMS week before menses, during the week-long menses, and during the recover, reenergize week after menses. That leaves a two day window of opportunity if "the kids are being good … the bills are paid, and the house is clean …"* for her and her partner to have intercourse. Hearing about this story, one of her friends retorted that her own "window of opportunity" was shut and that her shop was closed for business almost every day.

A 50-year-old female minister was surprised during a service with a slide show celebrating her faithful journey at the church over the last decade. After watching her slide show she said wistfully, "I haven't seen her for some time now." With time, your body will change. It is only natural that just as life goes through cycles, your body will go through cycles. Savor the change as a rite of passage to a new level of womanhood.

With time, you may feel a new sense of freedom and sexual intimacy as you enter your 40s and 50s. With your kids being older and more self-sufficient, your career under control, and you're getting closer to arriving at your life's goals, you may feel more confident, secure, and more attractive than you ever have before in your life.

As you arrive at the next level of womanhood, you will learn to love your changing body and appreciate its timeless beauty as you metamorphose to a new and better level in your life. And, at some point, you need to trust that your partner really does still find you desirable and very attractive—even with the lights on!

*Adapted from a Gibson Greeting Card referring to when life is good.

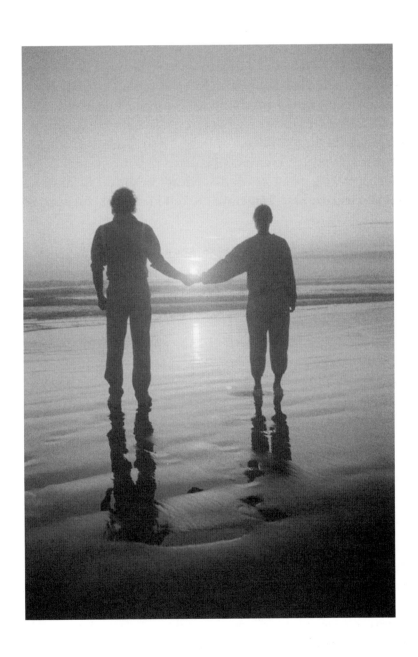

Question and Answers

Question #1: Where did my desire go?

Answer: If your sexual desire just seems to get up and leave you behind, feeling cold and left out, there is hope for you. There could be an emotional, physical, or medical cause for your lack of desire. The first thing you need to do is get a physical exam, pap, and pelvic scheduled. Together with your doctor you can begin to explore what might be the cause of your lack of desire. If you don't feel like you can talk to your doctor about this, write it out for your doctor to read, or ask a friend for a recommendation of a doctor who is easy to talk to and who can help guide you to find answers.

Question #2: What are some ideas to help get the spark and desire back?

Answer: "Sometimes when you look at your partner and he has started to look like the chair he always sits in, it is hard to get aroused."* When this happens, try to remember the things about him that attracted you to him in the first place, and allow yourself to fall in love with him all over again.

Remember that in order to show signs of intimacy it doesn't necessarily always have to be sexual. Great satisfaction can be achieved by the giving of your spirit. Some ideas include the following: have an intimate conversation just about the two of you, or leave affectionate notes on his pillow, in a briefcase or lunch box, or in lipstick on his mirror. Even an unexpected phone call to tell him "hi" and that you miss him can make him feel appreciated and loved. **Also, don't be afraid to show your partner what you prefer or what makes you feel the best. Remember to tell him what you want because he cannot read your mind!**

Question #3: Are there medications or drugs that can cause decreased desire or orgasms?

Answer: Yes! Sexual desire can be affected by antidepressants, heart or blood pressure medications, reflux medications, and anti-inflammatories. Drugs that decrease the ability to achieve orgasm include appetite suppressants, recreational drugs, antidepressants, sleep aids, and alcohol.

Question #4: What will the doctor be looking for on my physical exam?

Answer: Your doctor will examine the genital area to see if there are signs of scars, plaque, or lesions that could cause you discomfort during intercourse. Next, the vaginal opening will be examined for scarring, stricture, bleeding tissue, or discharge. Your doctor will also look at the inside of the vagina. Near menopause, the vagina will lose elasticity, have decreased lubrication, the walls will be thinner, and the secretions will become more basic than acidic; this pH change could cause increased infections. Your ovaries shrink in size, your uterus becomes smaller, and the uterus opening (the cervix) can become smaller. When doctors feel inside, they will be checking the bladder, uterus, or rectum. When these organs lose their muscle support, they cause discomfort, pressure, or constipation.

Question #5: Could there be a medical reason why I don't want relations with my partner?

Answer: There are some medical conditions that can cause decreased desire, excitement, or orgasm:** Hypoactive Sexual Desire Disorder is when there is a decrease, or absence, of sexual fantasies or sexual desire. Sexual Aversion Disorder is when there is a persistent avoidance of contact. Sexual Arousal Disorder is a continual lack of sexual excitement or lubrication during sexual stimulation thus causing discomfort during intercourse. Orgasmic Disorder is the persistent delay or lack of orgasm. Vaginismus is spasm of the vagina during intercourse. Also there is Dyspareunia or painful intercourse. There are multiple causes for these disorders. Some are fueled by life events, hormonal changes, relationship issues, or health issues. Treatment choices include understanding the cause, counseling, behavior modifications, sex therapy classes, or self help books. There are even companies like Slumber Parties Inc. that have in-home parties that sell FDA approved sugar-free, fat-free body butter, and other products to help educate you about your body and help with relationship maintenance.

*Adapted from Dr. Susan Johnson, M.D., Women's Health Symposium lecture, Oct. 23, 2001.
**Reference Diagnostic and Statistical Manual of Mental Disorders, Fourth Edition (DSM-IV).

Question #6: What are some treatment options that are available for women?

Answer: To restore vaginal moisture, the FDA has approved the use of estrogen. Estrogen topical choices include creams, vaginal rings, or vaginal tablets. Giving oral or topical estrogen will help to restore blood flow to the vagina and improve the pH of the secretion so that there are fewer infections. Also, over the counter lubricants can help with dryness. Testosterone has been shown to increase desire in some women. It is available by prescription. Viagra tests on women have shown little promise, so that option is out for now.

If there are adhesions, infections, or scarring, these can be treated by your doctor with medication or surgery. Urinary incontinence choices include Kegels, voiding retraining, or medications. Alternative medication options are not FDA approved or regulated. Buyer beware! Let you doctor know what you are considering, as it may be harmful to you or have a drug interaction with your current medicines.

Question #7: What is "normal" for sexual desire?

Answer: You and the standards that you set for yourself define "normal." If relations two times a month feels right for you, then it is right. If you perceive that sex equals intercourse, equals orgasm, equals happy ever after, you may be setting yourself and your partner up for disappointment. Your self-imposed pressure to perform or feel satisfied (or at least act like it) can leave you feeling challenged and exhausted. **Your goal should be to do what allows you to feel satisfied and reflects your values. If some nights that means cuddling on the couch together sharing a bowl of popcorn while watching your favorite movie, so be it! Do what you feel is right for you and leaves you feeling satisfied.**

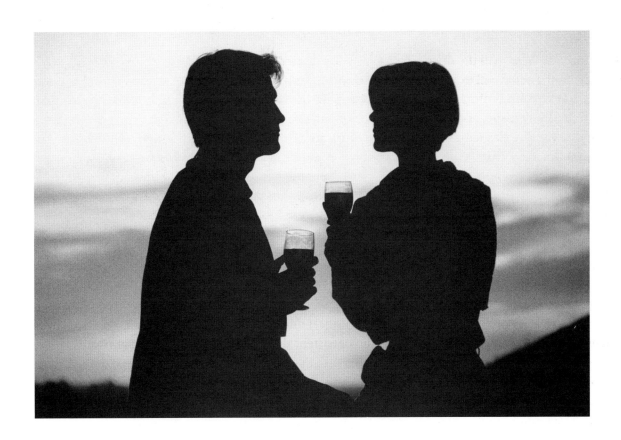

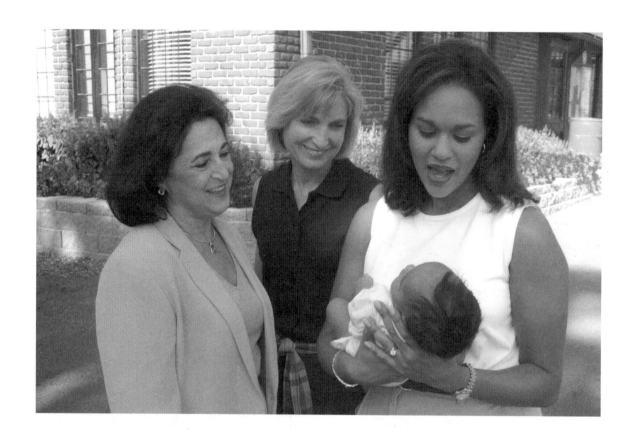

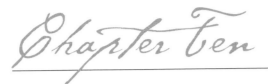

Chapter Ten

Yes, you can still get pregnant in this perimenopausal phase in your life. Just because you think you are too old to get pregnant, or you haven't had to use birth control pills in years, doesn't mean you can't get pregnant!

Chapter 10: Perimenopause

"I can't be pregnant—I'm too old" and "I can't be menopausal—I'm too young"

During perimenopause, your period can have a mind of its own. As your hormone levels start changing and your estrogen levels go up and down, surging and purging along, and your periods try to decide if they are coming or going. Perimenopause is the nine years before menopause. If you were once on a 28–35 day cycle, you may now have your period every 15–21 days (oh joy!), and if you once had a light flow and only a three day cycle, you may need stock in tampons because your flow could be heavy with clots and last for weeks—unbelievable!

Perimenopausal symptoms can include irregular menses, irritability, mood swings, food cravings, heart palpitations, sleep disturbances, weight changes, fatigue, memory changes, decreased sex drive, and hot flashes.

One of my mentors said perimenopause menses were like a car running out of gas—sputter, sputter, surge, lunge, sputter, sputter...finally coming to a halt. These irregular cycles can be frustrating and embarrassing, often catching you in locations and situations of bleeding occurrence when you would least expect a menses and are therefore completely unprepared. Changes in your menstrual cycle (and changes in your clothing) can be normal in the perimenopause phase of your life. However, any change that continues for more than two monthly cycles or any marked change in your cycle (box of tampons or pads used in just a few hours) should get you to your doctor's office. Some changes in your cycle need your doctor's help to diagnose and treat. Also, if you have spotting or bleeding after confirmed menopause, you may need to see your doctor as soon as possible.

The irregular menses cycle with perimenopause can be treated with a low dose birth control pill. It is felt that low dose birth control pills can help to treat the irregular cycles, hormonal shifts in mood, hot flashes, vaginal dryness, and help prevent pregnancy.

I recently attended a lecture in which the doctor was telling the story of a 51-year-old woman who had come in to see him to confirm menopause; this patient was certain she was in menopause with her symptoms of breast tenderness, tearfulness, and irregular cycles. The doctor proudly announced that before coming to give this lecture, he had just delivered this woman's bouncing baby boy. So, what the patient had interpreted as menopause symptoms at age 51, were really pregnancy symptoms!

One patient was having breast tenderness, moodiness, tearfulness, and irregular cycles and went to her OB/GYN for confirmation of menopause and was told these "menopausal" symptoms would disappear in the next nine months. Interestingly enough, she was told by the doctor's office that five other women had come in that same day to be confirmed with menopause, and they all left knowing that they were pregnant.

Yes, you can still get pregnant in the perimenopause phase of your life. Just because you think you are too old to get pregnant, or you haven't had to use birth control in years, doesn't mean you can't get pregnant! You definitely need to use protection against pregnancy in your 40s and 50s unless you have had a hysterectomy or confirmed menopause, or your husband has had a vasectomy. Or you, too, may be the person most surprised that your menopausal symptoms are actually a pregnancy.

If you do choose to take a low dose birth control pill for your perimenopause irregular menses, it may take up to three full months to finally regulate your cycle to a normal flow every 28 days.

If you are on the birth control pill now, how do you know when to stop the birth control or switch to actual hormone replacement therapy? If you are near 51 years of age, the average age of menopause, or are having menopausal-type symptoms, the best way is to stop your birth control pill for one to two weeks and have a follicle stimulating hormone (FSH) drawn to confirm that you have entered into menopause. If your FSH is greater than 30, it is probably okay to stop your birth control. This, then, would be the time you could stop the birth control pill or switch to short-term hormone replacement therapy—if the benefits outweigh the risks. For most women, the risks from taking long-term hormone replacement therapy outweigh the benefits, so other options to control menopausal symptoms may need to be considered.

If you switch to short-term hormone replacement therapy, and you start to have irregular cycles, you may need additional time for your body to adjust to the new hormone replacement therapy. If so, hormone replacement therapy that creates a menses cycle every 28 days may be your best option until your body's hormones are calmed down and your body is ready for the switch. After six months to one year of doing a menses 28-day cycling, you can then try to switch to short-term continuous hormone replacement therapy. After switching to short-term continuous hormone replacement therapy, any continuous spotting or menses may result in your needing further evaluation. This should be determined by your doctor.

Menopause (the last period of your life) should not be considered the beginning of the end. Instead, this is a new beginning for you; this is a chance for celebration. You can rejoice in your body taking you to the next phase of your life. No longer will there be only a two-day window of opportunity between PMS, premenstrual dysphoric syndrome, perimenopause, your menses, or post-period blues in which your family can safely approach you in a given month. Now your window can be wide open all the time, letting the beautiful blue sky, golden sunshine, and fresh air in for you to enjoy.

Tips for Perimenopause:

- Make healthy food and exercise choices; this can be a wonderful time in your life.
- In perimenopause your menses cycle may change.
- Be sure to still use some form of birth control in your perimenopause years.
- If you are having marked menopause hot flashes, or vaginal dryness, and/or your FSH is greater than 30, it may be time to consider short-term hormone replacement therapy (if the benefits outweigh the risks). For many women the risks of taking long-term HRT may outweigh the benefits so other options may need to be considered to control menopause symptoms.

Questions and Answers

Question #1: During my perimenopause years, how many irregular menstrual cycles should I have before seeing my doctor?

Answer: If you have more than two months of irregular menstrual bleeding, you may need to have further evaluation from your doctor. This could entail a simple pap smear, bimanual exam, or you may need an endometrial biopsy, ultrasound, or change in medicines.

Question #2: What is a low dose birth control pill?

Answer: A low dose birth control pill is normally around 20 micrograms of estrogen and it helps to protect against pregnancy; the birth control pill also helps create regular menses, decrease menstrual blood loss or anemia, and relieves menopause symptoms of hot flashes and vaginal dryness in addition to helping with other perimenopausal-type symptoms. Remember: taking an antibiotic may decrease the birth control pill's effectiveness in protecting against pregnancy.

Question #3: My mother is years into menopause and is still being cycled to have a period by her doctor. Is this okay?

Answer: After menopause there is little or no reason to have a menses. Remember, a menses function is simply to shed the lining of the uterus if an ovulated egg doesn't get fertilized. Your mother is postmenopausal and cannot release an egg because she is not ovulating after menopause; therefore, she does not need to have a menses to shed the uterus lining. Years ago, doctors observed that women seemed to be in a much better mood after their "blood letting" menses. Your mother has earned her right of passage into menopause and no longer needs to have a period. She should see her doctor about either being switched to a short-term continuous hormone replacement therapy that would avoid a menses, or discontinuing hormone replacement therapy because risks may outweigh the benefits.

Question #4: How do I know if it is a pregnancy or menopause symptoms if I am having irregular menses, breast tenderness, tiredness, tearfulness, etc.?

Answer: The best way is to see your doctor as soon as possible and have a pregnancy serum test drawn and/or a FSH level drawn, if deemed appropriate by your doctor. You doctor will then able to confirm if your symptoms are related to menopause or pregnancy.

Question #5: I have had menopausal-type symptoms, but still have a period—though somewhat irregular. When should an FSH be drawn, and at what point should hormone replacement therapy be considered?

Answer: If you are experiencing menopausal-type symptoms and/or having irregular menses and/or near the average age of 51 for menopause, it would be appropriate for you to get an FSH level drawn. An FSH test is not necessary to confirm menopause; being around 51 years of age and having no menses for six months with or without symptoms can be enough to confirm menopause. If your FSH level is greater than 30, you may consider taking short-term hormone replacement therapy if the benefits outweigh the risks. However, for most women, options other than hormone replacement therapy are available for the treatment of menopause symptoms.

If you are perimenopausal with irregular menses cycles, you can consider a low dose birth control pill which could protect you against pregnancy and regulate your menses. Low dose birth control pills have more estrogen than the standard hormone replacement therapy regimen. The standard hormone replacement therapy may not protect you against pregnancy if you are still ovulating and the hormone replacement therapy is given too early. Once your FSH is greater than 30 and your luteinizing hormone (LH) is greater than 30, it is felt that you are, at this time, protected against pregnancy.

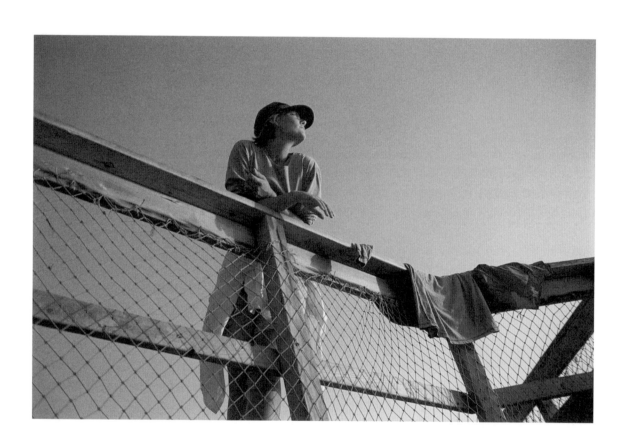

Chapter Eleven

How do you ever even begin to apologize to the entire world for what your hormones made you say or do the last two weeks? Let's face it, you can't be held responsible for your words or actions when your body has been taken hostage by your raging hormones.

Chapter 11: Perimenopause and PMS At the Same Time?

Most days, Sue is thoughtful and compassionate and has a great sense of humor that puts a smile on her face. Her days are filled with family, work, and extra curricular activities that involve her three children's sports and school activities. Sue is admired and respected by her friends and co-workers because of her coping and juggling skills and because she is able to get so many things completed in her 24-hour day with a smile on her face. Then, without even so much as a phone call to warn her, Sue's ugly and wicked identical twin sister arrives for a visit. Her twin sister never stays long, but she is horribly disruptive and nearly destroys Sue's life and balance when she does visit. Her twin sister is irritable, moody, and cries easily. She snaps at people for the tiniest of reasons. Sometimes, Sue cannot even believe the words that come out of her twin's mouth. After all, the human tongue can be a dangerous weapon; the words a tongue speaks can destroy another person as much as any physical weapon. Sue's ugly twin sister leaves a path of destruction behind her wherever she goes. You can always tell where she has been—just follow the path of wounded. The days her twin sister arrives for visits, Sue thinks she is completely losing her mind.

If the truth were to be told, Sue actually doesn't even have a twin sister. But who or what else could explain her almost out-of-body experience that happens every month? Her monthly personality change seems to arrive without warning and when it leaves, her life is in shambles. Sue is left feeling completely overwhelmed and betrayed by her own mind and body.

Behind Sue's blue eyes there was a hurricane roaring. The internal hurricane started with a little whirlwind of air swirling in the middle of her menstrual cycle, stirring up her hormone balance. It gathered momentum and force into a huge, raging, roaring, unpredictable storm of emotion before her menses were to start. Even though her family, friends, and co-workers knew Hurricane Sue was starting to stir and would be arriving soon, their efforts of self-preservation—leaving the area and boarding up their emotions—could not protect them at times from the wrath of Hurricane Sue. Somewhere deep inside, Sue knew that there was the peaceful, calm eye of the storm; soon Hurricane Sue would pass, and the seas would once again be peaceful and harmonious.

If you suffer from premenstrual syndrome, you know your emotional life can be unpredictable. One of my friends suffers terribly from PMS. For her birthday, we found the perfect card for her. It was a woman decked out in military gear on the front and on the inside it says "I have PMS beware—I am armed and dangerous."

One of my patients stated that her boyfriend told her, after years of trying to avoid her during her PMS time, he finally figured out that he should harness her argumentative, out-of-my-way-I-am-going-to-get-what-I-want-don't-mess-with-me PMS attitude; he would take her with him at those times when he needed to negotiate the best price for a new car, business contracts, and the like.

Another patient was in for her physical, and mentioned that she had been struggling with PMS symptoms the week before each period. On one particularly rough PMS day, she said that she was fed up with the frustration at home and announced with defiance, "I am leaving to go shopping!" Her partner, not usually much of a shopper, said, "I am going with you." My patient snapped at him, "Why?" Her partner tactfully responded, "To protect the store employees!"

After having lived through another PMS cycle, most of us look back over the last two weeks of our cycle and wonder what it was that possessed our bodies and made us say and do all of those things that you would have never said or done if not in a PMS cycle. How do you ever even *begin* to apologize to the entire world for what your hormones made you say or do over the last two weeks? Let's face it, you can't be held responsible for your own words or actions when your body is being taken hostage by your raging hormones.

One way to be more responsible for your actions is to be able to predict when your emotional hurricane may be arriving. Making a graph or chart for three months can be both enlightening and empowering. After graphing your emotions, signs, and symptoms for three months, you can predict—almost to the day—when you should avoid certain activities. If day 20 of your cycle is the day you usually feel overwhelmed, irritable, and bloated, this is probably not the day to have your in-laws over for that special dinner. It may be better to follow your upswing recovery time on your cycle and have them over on day 10. Both you, and your in-laws, will be glad you did.

What exactly is PMS—other than the time during your monthly cycle you say **P**lease let the real **M**e **S**tand up? Premenstrual syndrome symptoms occur approximately five days before your menses and resolve, or are relieved, four days into your menses. **You probably have PMS if the symptoms have reoccurred over the last three menstrual cycles. According to the American College of GYN diagnostic criteria for PMS, you must report one of the following symptoms during the five days before each period in each of the three prior menstrual cycles: depression, angry outbursts, irritability, anxiety, confusion, social withdrawal, breast tenderness, abdominal bloating, headache, swelling of extremities, water retention, or food cravings.**

What exactly causes PMS? It all starts in your brain with the neurotransmitters' messages sent to your ovaries and uterus, by your brain, to increase or decrease the production of estrogen and progesterone. Prostaglandin levels also play a role in PMS. After your menses cycle is complete, your body starts to make increased levels of estrogen to prepare an egg for release from your ovary. The increased estrogen level relieves your PMS symptoms. The increased estrogen gives you a sense of harmony and balance. At this time, as your estrogen level is increasing, you have less progesterone. Then at mid-cycle, usually day 14, when you ovulate (ovulation is when your ovary releases the prepared egg) your body decreases its amount of estrogen production and increases your progesterone production in order to prepare your uterus or womb for a fertilized egg. Your body is sensitive to the increased progesterone and this is why you often will start to notice PMS symptoms such as breast swelling and tenderness, irritability, and mood swings after your ovulate. If the egg is not fertilized, your progesterone level decreases and your body sloughs off the inner prepared womb tissue in the form of a menses; the womb isn't needed now because the egg wasn't fertilized. When your body decreases its production of progesterone, you have a menses and this is when you finally feel relief from your PMS symptoms for the next two-plus weeks, or at least until your mid cycle or ovulation time. If your body has an imbalance of prostaglandin E, you may have increased PMS symptoms. It is important to take one multivitamin daily and eat well. You need to eat foods that include magnesium, linoleic acid, vitamins B3, B6, C, and zinc.

What if your PMS symptoms seem beyond the listed symptoms and seem to completely be out of your control? Do you even have symptoms that include homicidal and suicidal thoughts? If so, you may be suffering from the severe form of PMS called premenstrual dysphonic disorder (PMDD). PMS and PMDD usually occur after ovulation (day 14 of cycle) and during the luteal (increased progesterone phase) before your menses. **PMDD, in addition to having the above mentioned PMS symptoms, also includes self-doubt, decreased efficiency in tasks, decreased concentration, decreased ability to complete tasks, increased distraction, negative thoughts, and hostility towards other people. With PMS you can have mild, moderate, or severe symptoms. If you have severe PMS symptoms, it is called PMDD.**

If you have a menstruation cycle, there is a 25 percent chance you will have some level of PMS. Three to five percent of the time it will be severe enough to be classified as PMDD. With overlapping symptoms, how do you ever tell the difference between PMDD and depression? **With PMDD, your symptoms resolve within days of the start of your menses. With PMDD you will also have symptoms like bloating and breast tenderness that don't occur with depression.**

The new serotonin reuptake inhibitors work well for both depression and PMDD. Phases in your life that cause hormonal shifts such as ovulation, pregnancy, and menopause help to decrease PMDD and PMS symptoms. I know a women and her husband who are counting the probable number of cycles and PMS swings until her menopause. She is 45 years of age. The average age of menopause is 51.4. If their calculations are right, she has 96 cycles to go until menopause—then no more PMS. They can't wait!

Do women who think their irritable mood swings are because of PMS actually have it? No, not always. That is why it is best to do the PMS calendar for three cycles. You may, instead, be suffering from chronic depression. If you have PMS, do you have to be treated? No. If you find that your symptoms are severe enough that you cannot function at home, school, work, or socially, then you need to consider treatment. **What are your treatment choices? Well, first things first. You have to start taking better care of yourself. That means you need to eat a nutritious diet, sleep seven to eight hours nightly, and exercise for 30 minutes daily. Watch your salt and fatty food intake, and decrease the amount of alcohol you consume.** You might also consider taking a serotonin reuptake inhibitor. One of the new serotonin reuptake inhibitors, called Sarafem, can be taken starting on day 14 of your cycle and be continued until your period starts. Then, the medicine can be stopped. This works well for both PMS and PMDD.

While most days you can conceal or camouflage your PMS/PMDD mood swings while at work, school, or in social situations, it is your husband and children that usually end up taking the brunt of your PMS hormonal mood swings. Your husband and kids would probably be relieved if you would start to take better care of yourself. You may need to consider trying a serotonin reuptake inhibitor during your PMS symptoms. One of my friends said her son told her, "Mom it used to be you would have PMS only a few days a month. Now it seems like you have it every day!"

Despite feeling overwhelmed, out of control, and like you are losing your mind during your PMS symptoms, you can be in better control of your PMS mood swings with a little help from your diet, exercise, and possibly medicine. There is some thought that vitamin E, vitamin B6, calcium, relaxation therapy, coping skill technique, massage therapy, or anti-inflammatories may help decrease your PMS/PMDD symptoms. Research is still ongoing in this area, and there is not yet any convincing evidence that any of these treatments work. When considering your choices for treating PMS, remember: just one good daily multivitamin is sufficient. Taking additional vitamins, herbs, and supplements may be harmful or toxic to your health.

Instead of being armed and dangerous with PMS symptoms, be armed and empowered with knowledge to control your PMS symptoms. You can try to control your hormonal swings by charting the cycle of your symptoms. By predicting that on day 18 you are always irritable, you can schedule that important meeting or dinner on your in-control days. Eat a well-balanced, nutritious diet, rest seven to eight hours a night, drink 64 ounces of water a day, quit smoking, watch your salt intake (keep it less than three grams a day), and exercise by doing your favorite workout for 30 minutes a day.

Tips for PMS:

- Use a PMS chart for three months to track daily emotions and symptoms to confirm PMS.
- How do you know it is only PMS? All signs and symptoms stop a few days after the start of your menses.
- Treatments include: better nutrition; decreasing caffeine, nicotine, and animal fats; increasing vegetable oils; exercising, sleeping, drinking 64 ounces of water, taking one daily multivitamin, and avoiding salty and fatty foods.
- Avoid scheduling stressful activities on your increased symptomatic PMS days.
- Consider a serotonin reuptake inhibitor as your life buoy during your PMS emotional hurricane days.

Questions and Answers

Question #1: What exactly causes PMS?
Answer: It all starts in your brain with neurotransmitter messages sending signals to your ovary and uterus to increase and decrease the production of estrogen and progesterone. When your estrogen levels are up, you feel more harmonious and in balance. When your progesterone levels are up, you often will have breast swelling, tenderness, irritability, mood swings, and other typical PMS-type symptoms.

Question #2: My PMS symptoms seem to markedly interfere with my work and relationships, but I don't want to take medicine. Any other suggestions?
Answer: Avoid scheduling activities with your loved ones or important work meetings on your predictably worst PMS days. Schedule your most important meetings and events on your upswing harmonious days. Try rose hip tea to calm, a warm bath in the evening, or massage therapy. Take well-deserved vacation days off. Do something special to pamper yourself during these times.

Question #3: I did the charting and it seems I have symptoms every day. Is this still PMS?
Answer: With PMS, you may have breast tenderness and swelling included in your symptoms. With PMS you will also have complete relief of your symptoms for at least a brief time after your menses starts. Depression symptoms do not include breast tenderness and swelling; so, if there is no relief of your other symptoms (even with a menstruation cycle), you may have depression. Talk to your physician about lifestyle changes that will allow you to function well and live your life to the fullest.

Question #4: It is possible to have both PMS and depression?
Answer: Absolutely. Fortunately, the new serotonin reuptake inhibitors will help the symptoms for both PMS and depression. It has not been proven whether or not taking a birth control pill will help, it could, in fact, exacerbate PMS symptoms. Your doctor is waiting to help you. Make the call. You don't have to suffer with PMS or depression symptoms any longer. You can live your life to the fullest each and every single day.

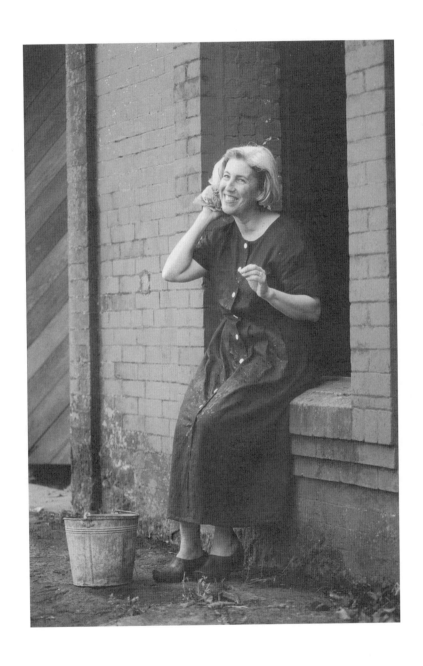

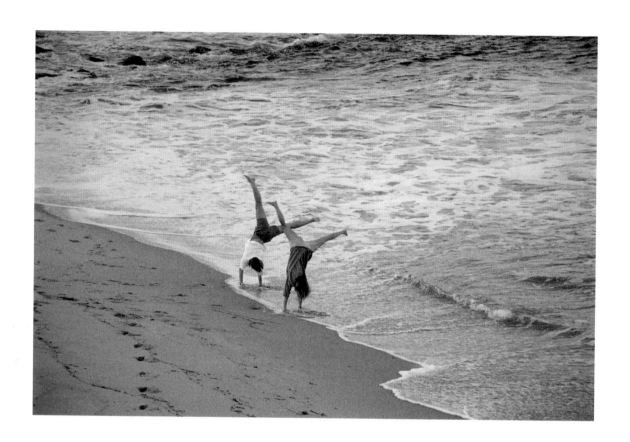

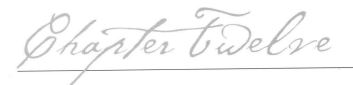

Chapter Twelve

A normal pap smear result should say, "normal." Your doctor's office should mail or call you with your results. If you do not receive your results, DO NOT assume that "no news is good news!"

Chapter 12: Pap Smears
Making Sense of Your Results

In all of the years that I have performed pap smears, I have yet to have a patient come in for a pap smear jumping for joy and clapping her hands singing, "I can't wait to have my pap smear done today. I have been looking forward to this all week long and this will be the highlight of my day!" and saying, "Let's get started," jumping anxiously into the stirrups.

Au contraire! Most of the time the patients are tightly tied into their examination gown with arms tightly wrapped around their chests. Their arms act as a physical barrier to block their body, and their legs are tightly crossed as they suspiciously eye the cold metal stirrups and speculum. All the while, they are having flashbacks of previous paps. They meekly utter, "Do we have to do this?"

Pap smears were designed by Dr. Papanicolaou as a way to detect cervical cancer. The cervix is the opening of your uterus. (The cervix is the hole from which the baby comes out of the uterus). Since the time pap smear screens were started, cervical cancer detection has dramatically increased and lives have been saved. Pap smear screens should be started when you are 18 years old or have become sexually active—whichever comes first in your life. If you are on birth control pills, or have had previously abnormal pap smears, you may need to get a pap smear performed at least once a year. If your pap smears have always been completely normal, and you are not taking a birth control pill, you may be able to go one to every three years for pap smears.

As you enter perimenopause and menopause you may think that just because you are done having children you are "done" with that part of your body. However, despite your rationale in trying to talk yourself out of having your lovely stirrup and speculum event performed, you may still need to have a pap smear performed.

And, remember, the pap smear is only to look for cervical cancer. It is not used to diagnose vaginal, uterus, or ovary cancer. With your pap, a pelvic (and possibly a rectal exam) needs to be done. During the pelvic exam, the doctor examines the genital area looking for tumors, bumps, and abnormalities. The doctor then examines the vaginal area looking for any infection or abnormalities. The doctor places her hand inside the vagina to feel the uterus' contour, shape, and position. During the pelvic exam, if you are postmenopausal, your ovaries should not be able to be felt. If you doctor is able to feel your ovaries and you are postmenopausal, you need further investigation of your ovaries with an ultrasound, cat scan, or biopsy.*

Your pap, pelvic, rectal, and breast exams can be preformed by an OB/GYN doctor, family practice physician, physician assistant, or nurse practitioner. If you are done having children and are still seeing your OB/GYN, you may want to switch to having your pap smears done by your family doctor.

A normal pap smear result should say, "normal." Your doctor's office should mail or call you with your results. If you do not hear or receive your results DO NOT assume that "no news is good news!" If you haven't received your results within three weeks of your pap exam, call your doctor for your results.

The best time to have a pap smear is one week after your menses. If you are in menopause and have had normal pap smears, most any time of the month is okay. It is best to not have anything in your vagina one week prior to your pap smear. This includes gel, creams, or medicines. Pap slide technologists have a limit to how many pap slides they can read in a day. Having any type of vaginal discharge such as sperm, mucous, or menses is like asking the pap slide technologist to look through a muddy window shield and tell you—with confidence—that they don't see any abnormal cells on your slide. If you are having cervical discharge, you might ask your doctor to use a large cervical swab to clean away the vaginal or cervical discharge or consider rescheduling.

If you have had your cervix removed by a hysterectomy for non-cancer reasons, it has been determined that you may not need pap smears performed. If you have had a hysterectomy for cancer reasons, you may need a yearly pap, taking cells from the vaginal cuff (mucosal ridge of vagina where uterus was before surgery).

How do you make sense out of your pap smear results and determine what you are to do next? The "How to Interpret Your Pap Smear Results" chart may help you to better understand your pap results.

The important thing to remember is to get your pap done every year to every three years if all paps have been normal and you are not taking a birth control pill. Remember to call early as you may have to wait up to six months for a pap smear when you call to schedule.

Think of your yearly pap as a great time to discuss your health questions with your doctor and to get good health tip updates on prevention ideas that are customized to your lifestyle.

*According to research there is no screening method for ovarian cancer; Serum CA-125 and ultrasound tests only help to diagnose the disease and are not for screening purposes. If you have a family history of ovarian cancer there may be genetic testing your doctor can advise.

Tips for Pap Smears:

- Regularly scheduled paps are a must. If all pap smears have been normal, then having a pap smear every one to three years may be satisfactory. If you are on birth control or have had abnormal paps, then you may need yearly pap smears.
- The best time for your pap to be scheduled is one week after your menses.
- If pap is abnormal, schedule right away for further intervention (see "How to Interpret Your Pap Smear Results" chart in this chapter).

Question and Answers

Question #1: Is there anything that can be done about those cold metal speculums?
Answer: Fortunately, a newer plastic speculum is available that may feel warmer to you than metal. Some exam tables have a warming drawer, and some doctors use a heating pad or their hands to warm the speculum for you. Ask your doctor about the available options.

Question #2: I'm not sexually active and have never had kids, do I still need paps?
Answer: Although, technically, your risk for having an abnormal pap is lower because you haven't been exposed to viruses that can be transmitted sexually, you may still need a pap smear. It is a good idea to schedule routine paps; this is a way for you to be proactive and to stay on top of your health. Again, if your pap has always been normal and you are not on birth control pills, you may be able to get a pap every one to three years.

Question #3: I have had a hysterectomy (uterus removed) do I still need paps?
Answer: If your uterus was removed for non-cancer reasons you may not require a pap (remember a pap looks for cervical cancer, and your cervix was removed with the hysterectomy). However, depending on your age, a yearly pelvic, rectal, breast exam, and mammogram should still be scheduled.* If you had a hysterectomy due to cancer then you should consider getting a vaginal cuff test (similar to pap test) done to look at the cells where the cervix used to be.

Question #4: When is the best time to schedule a pap?
Answer: If you could schedule a pap for next year as you check out at the medical reception desk after this year's pap, that would be great. Remember to try to schedule your pap one week after your menses. (Yes, that can be tricky, especially if your cycle isn't regular.) There should be nothing placed in the vagina for one week prior to your pap. Creams, lotions, gels, tampons, intercourse, and infections can alter your results.

Question #5: At what age can I stop getting paps?
Answer: At one time it was felt that at age 75 you could stop getting paps because you had reached the average age of life expectancy. Now, with a preventive lifestyle and modern medicine you can expect to live well into your 80s. Although as you age your cervical cancer risk goes down, your risk for other diseases may go up. So, a regularly scheduled **physical exam** can be a wonderful opportunity to discuss your health. Remember, it has been said that health is all about "PREVENT-DETECT-TREAT" to ensure a bright and robust future.

Question #6: What types of pap smears are available?
Answer: The current standard pap is performed by using a small wooden or plastic spatula. It is rubbed across the cervical cells on top of the cervix. Then a tiny round tip brush (cytobrush) is twirled once inside the cervix to get the cells inside of the cervix. The spatula and cytobrush are gently and quickly wiped across a slide and then sprayed with a cell preservative and sent to a lab to be analyzed. The newest type of pap is called "thin" prep pap test; your part of the pap will seem the same, but the doctor will handle the cells differently. The doctor will use the same technique to obtain the cervix cells, but instead of wiping the cells onto a slide, the doctor will put the cells into a small liquid preservative filled jar; the jar is sent to the lab where the cells are then placed onto a slide. At the lab, the jar liquid is run through a filter that washes off any mucous, debris, or blood from the cervix cells. The advantage of the thin prep pap test is that it removes a lot of artifact and debris so the technologist can read your slide more accurately. The thin prep liquid can be stored for three weeks and used to analyze for Human Papillomavirus (HPV). The liquid prep pap test is more expensive and not all labs are equipped yet to process the jars. However, the liquid prep, or other newer methods of doing paps, may start to be the way of the future for pap smear collection if the cost becomes more affordable and more labs are equipped to process the newer methods.

*See "Health Maintenance Guidelines" chart in Chapter 2

Question #7: What does an abnormal pap with a low-grade intraepithelial lesion really mean?

Answer: It means that your pap smear showed a mild abnormality. Each year, two to three million American women receive pap smears that show mildly abnormal results. These abnormal cells are then called atypical squamous cells of undetermined significance (ASC-US) or low-grade squamous intraepithelial lesions (LSIL). AS-CUS is usually caused by cell changes due to inflammation, irritation, or repair.

If your pap reads AS-CUS, then your pap should be repeated in three to six months, or a colposcopy exam should be considered to make sure your cervical cells have returned to normal. If your pap says ASC-H, then they cannot exclude a higher grade squamous intraepithelial lesion (ASC-H), so you may need a colpscopy with a biopsy. If your pap results state LSIL, this may require a colonoscopy and a biopsy. These cell changes are usually due to a virus called Human Papillomavirus (HPV). Approximately 60 percent of the time LSIL will regress back to normal cells without any treatment, and the pap smears will return to normal. However, up to eleven percent of the time there will be progression of HPV to a high grade lesion or cancer. If your pap states LSIL, you may need to get an HPV test to see if your lesion is HPV positive or negative. If you are HPV positive, then a colpscopy, biopsy, and possible treatment may need to be done. If you are HPV negative, you should repeat your paps every three months until three normal consecutive paps are obtained. Then you may need to have a pap every six months for the next year. If all your paps remain normal, you can return to a yearly pap smear schedule. If the repeat paps continue to be abnormal you should talk to your doctor about proceeding to colpscopy, biopsy, or possible treatment.

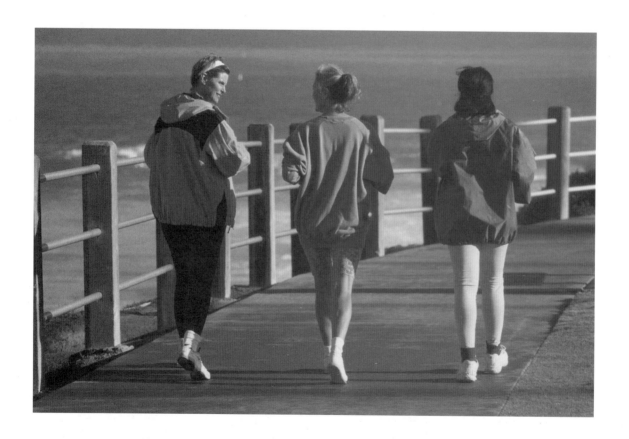

How to Interpret Your Pap Smear Results
Based on the new Bethesda, Maryland 2001 system

	Action
Specimen Adequacy (could the technician read the slide)	
Unsatisfactory for evaluation	Need to repeat your pap ASAP to keep on a yearly schedule
Satisfactory for evaluation	Move on to "Interpretation/Results" section

Interpretation/ Results
Here technician describes the cells seen on your slide:

	Action
Negative for intraepithelial lesion or malignancy: "normal"	Repeat routine pap

Negative for intraepithelial lesion or malignancy
No cancer cells seen but technician did notice:

	Action
Organisms like candida (yeast) bacterial vaginosis (gardnerella), herpes cells, Trichomonas cells	Need treatment advice. May need repeat pap
Or reactive or reparative cells caused from inflammation (tampon use, recent intercourse, menses), radiation, or IUD use	Repeat pap in 6 months
Or cell changes from a hysterectomy or atrophy (aging cells)	Repeat routine pap

Epithelial Cell Abnormalities
Technician saw unusual changes in your cells:
Squamous= vagina or cervix, Glandular=uterus

Squamous cells 4 types: atypical, low grade, high grade, or squamous cell carcinoma

Atypical squamous cells (ASC)

	Action
Undetermined significance (ASC-US) or,	Repeat pap in 3-6 months
Cannot exclude HSIL (ASC-H)	May need colposcopy, biopsy
Low grade squamous intraepithelial lesion (LSIL) Surface cells show a change that may progress to high grade lesion or cancer. Usually caused by HPV. Formerly known as mild dysphasia or CIN 1.	May need colposcopy, biopsy. Repeat pap every 3 months until 3 in a row normal, repeat every 6 months for a year, then routine paps if normal
High grade squamous intraepithelial lesion (HSIL) Very concerning cell changes seen that may progress to cancer. Formerly known as moderate, severe dysphasia or carcinoma in-situ, or CIN2, CIN3, CIS.	NOW, see a doctor for colpscopy, biopsy, and possible treatment. Repeat pap every 3 months until 3 in in a row normal, repeat every 6 months for a year, then routine paps if normal.
Squamous cell carcinoma=cervix cancer Cells change from normal-atypical-low grade-high grade-cancer	See a specialist NOW for treatment

Glandular Cells
Technician saw abnormal cells from inside cervix or uterus.
Four types:

	Action
Atypical: endocervical, endometrial, or glandular (not specific for cancer) **Atypical:** endocervical, or glandular (concerning changes in cell seen) **Endocervical adenocarcinoma insitu-:** (cancer of the cervix) **Adenocarcinoma:** endocervical, endometrial, or extrauterine cancer	All abnormal glandular paps need to **see doctor** for biopsy, colposcopy. Treat if needed, repeat pap every 3 months until 3 are normal, then repeat every 6 months for a year, then routine paps if normal.

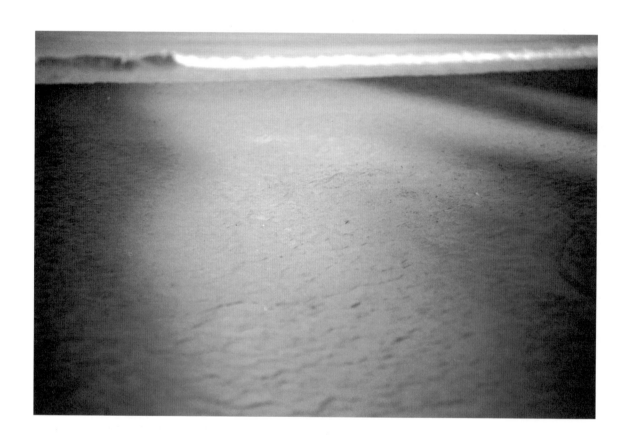

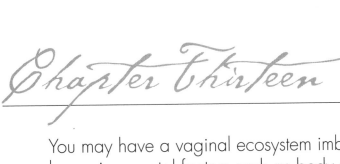

Chapter Thirteen

You may have a vaginal ecosystem imbalance caused by environmental factors such as body stress, or an illness that creates an imbalance of your vaginal flora mucosa that may cause you discomfort.

Chapter 13: Vaginal Dryness Relief at Last

In the perimenopausal and menopausal years, vaginal dryness is often caused by decreased estrogen production. As we age, our ovaries decrease their production of estrogen which results in a decreased level of vaginal moisture. With decreased vaginal moisture, you can notice vaginal or vulvar itching or painful intercourse. Vaginal dryness can be a result of hormonal changes in the pH balance of your vagina, which then can lead to an overgrowth of normal flora causing increased urinary tract infections and burning with urination.

You have different microorganisms that normally live in peace and harmony in the vaginal area. If there is a pH or electrolyte disturbance in this area, you can have an overgrowth of the normal flora, such as yeast, lactobacilli, or gardnerella that then causes symptoms of "yeast infection," or "vaginosis." You may feel that the discharge, burning, or itching caused by these overgrowths are too embarrassing to talk to your doctor about. Don't be shy in telling your doctor about your vaginal discomfort, discharge, or concerns. You don't have to continue to suffer or be uncomfortable. Tell your doctor where it itches and what is bothering you so she/he can help you.

Any continual vaginal itch, burning, dryness, or discomfort with intercourse or tampons, increased number of urinary tract infections, or chronic overgrowths of yeast or lactobacilli should be investigated by your doctor. Schedule a pelvic exam with your doctor to look at the vulvar and vaginal area. It may be necessary to do a vaginal culture or urinalysis to confirm the cause for your discomfort.

If it is confirmed that a decreased estrogen level is the cause of your dry vaginal symptoms, you can choose from several different treatment options to restore the moisture. You can choose lubricants to add moisture. Or, if you are postmenopausal, you can increase vaginal moisture by restoring estrogen using an oral pill, vaginal estrogen creams, suppositories or estrogen vaginal rings. Vaginal creme, suppository, or ring estrogen may be absorbed less easily into your blood system than oral estrogen. Vaginal estrogen does not seem to have the same effect of increased triglycerides as oral estrogen; however, vaginal estrogen does not seem to help with hot flashes or prevent osteoporosis. Other options to help when low estrogen causes vaginal dryness include using lubricants, or phytoestrogen products like soy, black cohosh, or red clover.

What if you are in your 30s and 40s and your estrogen level is normal, and you are experiencing these symptoms? You may have a vaginal ecosystem imbalance caused by environmental factors such as body stress, or an illness that creates an imbalance of your vaginal flora mucosa. The vaginal ecosystem, which was in perfect peace and harmony, is now at an imbalance, and you may develop an overgrowth of yeast or lactobacilli in your vagina; this can cause itching or discharge symptoms.

The vulvar and vaginal areas are very sensitive to any emotional, chemical, or body change. That is why when you are ill and receive an antibiotic you may get a "yeast infection." These really are not infections but are merely overgrowths of your normal flora that take place when you are ill or your body is stressed. The vaginal ecosystem pH gets out of balance when you are ill or taking an antibiotic, and the normally benign vaginal yeast can overgrow like a weed, causing a yeast overgrowth or "infection."

Because these overgrowths of yeast are so common and are relatively safe to treat, most treatment products are now available over the counter. If you prefer a pill for your "yeast infection," ask your doctor about getting one pill of oral medicine called Diflucan to treat your yeast overgrowth. Should you continue to get "yeast infections," or you have vaginal discharge that does not seem to go away, then you may need to get a pelvic exam and a vaginal culture to help identify and diagnose what may be causing your symptoms.

If your vulvar or vaginal areas are sensitive, R. Galask, M.D. and Mary Fraser, R.N. from the University of Iowa Hospitals and Clinics OB/GYN Nursing Division have prepared an excellent handout on guidelines for vulvar skin care. I have found that the suggestions below are exceptionally helpful for my patients and have proven to stand the test of time in assisting with keeping healthy vulvar and vaginal areas. The following are their recommendations:

- For laundry, use a mild enzyme-free soap such as Woolite Gentle or All Free and Clear. Remember to use only 1/3 to 1/2 the suggested amount because your undergarments may not need as much soap as is listed on the soap bottle.
- Do not use fabric dryer sheets or fabric softener.
- For clothing, wear white all-cotton underpants (not nylon) with a cotton crotch. (Jockey for Her and Hanes Her Way are two brands.)
- Avoid panty hose.
- Avoid tight fitting clothes and clothes made of synthetic, polyester, nylon, etc.
- Remove wet bathing and exercise clothing as soon as possible.
- For bathing and hygiene, avoid bath soaps, lotions, and gels that contain perfumes and can irritate the vulvar area.
- Choose products that say "mild" such as Dove Unscented, Neutrogena, or Cetaphil.
- Avoid bubble baths, bath salts, and scented oils.
- Do not scrub the vulvar area with a washcloth. Washing with your hand is good enough for cleaning. Pat dry (rather than rub) with a towel.
- Avoid douching.
- Try sitz baths with baking soda to help soothe the vulvar area with itching and burning.
- Avoid use of deodorized pads and tampons.
- Small amounts of A&D Ointment may be applied to your vulvar area.
- Try not to shave the vulvar area.
- Use white, unscented toilet paper.
- Avoid all feminine hygiene sprays, perfumes, and adult and baby wipes.
- If there is burning with urination, try pouring lukewarm water over the vulvar area.
- For larger women with chronic dampness, keep the area dry—consider using a hair dryer with a cool setting. Also consider using Gold Bond Powder.
- For vaginal dryness with intercourse, use a small pad of pure vegetable oil such as Crisco. Rinse away the Crisco with water after intercourse.

Questions and Answers

Question #1: I don't seem to have any of the previously mentioned symptoms. Do I still need to follow the good vulvar and vaginal hygiene regimen?
Answer: Everyone should probably follow this medically sound advice for good vulvar/vaginal hygiene. If perfumes, powders, and wearing unique underwear doesn't seem to bother you, grab the glitter lotion and thong underwear and strut your stuff.

Question #2: Can't a girl still have some fun while following vulvar recommendations?
Answer: Sure, you can still have some fun and feel sexy. You can enjoy the fun underwear and use gels, and lotions. You just might have to limit the exposure time your skin has to these products and wash the lotions, gels, etc., off and change undergarments after...

Question #3: Do I need to be routinely checked for vaginal "things?"
Answer: You should probably have a vaginal pelvic and pap every year if you are sexually active and/or on birth control pills. You might need to have a pelvic, pap, and vaginal exam sooner if symptoms warrant further investigation. That way, any vaginal changes (unnoticed discharge or skin changes) can be diagnosed early and (if needed) treated aggressively. Your doctor has been trained to see any worrisome signs and will get the appropriate cultures and treatment for you.

Question #4: What is the best thing to do for that embarrassing vaginal itch?
Answer: First, be checked by your physician to determine the cause. If the itching is allergic (chemical dyes, perfumes, etc.) follow the University of Iowa suggestions in this chapter. If it is purely dryness, try Vagisil Cream, K-Y Jelly, Vaseline, or—yes—even Crisco (it's not just for the kitchen anymore!). If the itch is due to severe dryness from decreased estrogen production, you many need to work with your doctor to choose from estrogen replacement therapy options such as vaginal creams, suppositories, or rings.

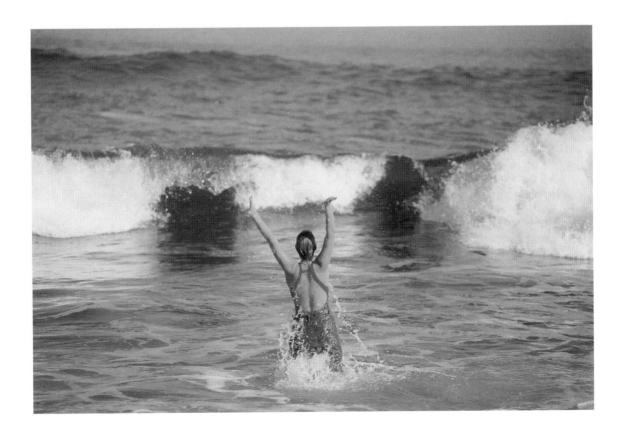

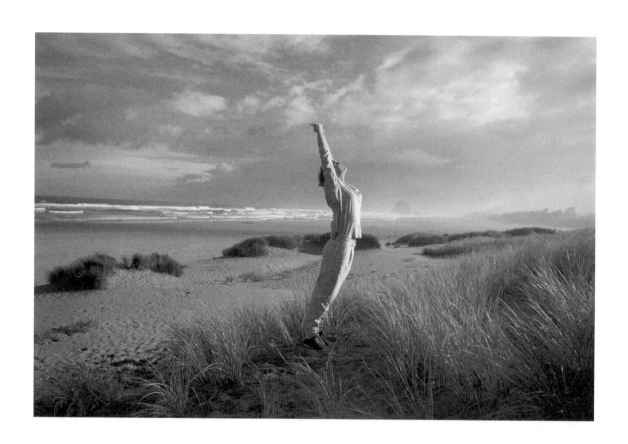

Your chance of getting breast cancer if you live into
your 90s, is one in eight. Your risk for breast cancer
increases as you age.

Chapter 14: *Breast Health*
Examine Your Risks

Your chance of getting breast cancer in your lifetime, if you live into your 90s, is 1 in 8. In other words, out of eight women that you know, one will get breast cancer in her lifetime. Before age 54, your risk is 1 in 54. Out of 24 women diagnosed with breast cancer, one person will die of the disease. The risk of developing breast cancer increases after you are 40 years old.

What are your risks for developing breast cancer? Please take the following survey to identify your risks:

Your Personal Risk Survey for Breast Cancer

	YES	NO
• Did your menses start when you were younger than age 11?	___	___
• Did you have your first pregnancy after age 30?	___	___
• Did you go into menopause after 52 years of age?	___	___
• Have your mother, sister, or daughter been diagnosed with breast cancer?	___	___
• Have you had breast cancer?	___	___
• Have you had breast atypical hyperplasia?	___	___
• Have you used birth control pills?	___	___
• Have you used estrogen hormone replacement therapy for over 4 years?	___	___
• Are you over 50 years of age?	___	___
• Are you 20 pounds overweight or more?	___	___
• Do you have the BRCA1 or the BRCA2 gene?	___	___

The more "yes" answers given, the higher your risk. Remember: aging is a risk factor, so all women have at least one risk factor.

Note: You can go to http://bcra.nci.nih.gov/brc/ to evaluate your individual risk of breast cancer over a five year period, and over a lifetime (to age 90). Another source for breast cancer information is the Cancer Information Service: 1-800-4-CANCER.

Screening for breast lumps

Remarkably, eighty percent of the time you will find a breast lump on your own by doing a self-breast exam. Anytime that you feel a breast lump that feels different than your other breast lumps (if it is irregularly shaped, non-mobile, you notice skin dimpling, nipple retraction, or discharge) you should be examined by your doctor. Anytime you feel a lump that concerns you, see your doctor.

If you have breast implants, your breast exam can be challenging., but you should still try to follow the screening recommendations. The more familiar you become with how your breasts feel (with or without implants), the better able you will be to detect a change in your breast tissue. Early breast cancer and some types of breast cancer are hard to detect.

There are three basic ways to help you screen for breast lumps. These include a self breast exam, a professional breast exam in a clinic, and a mammogram. A mammogram can pick up a small breast cancer before you can feel it. If you are at higher risk for breast cancer, you may benefit from a screening by mammogram in your 30s or 40s.

How to do a self breast exam

Do your breast exam once a month, one week after your menses. If you are menopausal, examine yourself the first day of each month. Lie flat on your bed, place a small pillow or rolled towel under the shoulder of the breast you are about to examine, and raise your arm above your head (this elevates the breast for a better exam). Use the flat part of the index and middle finger of the opposite hand to palpate the elevated breast. Your examining fingertips should gently make a small circle on the superficial top skin. While staying in the same spot, gently circle—pressing deeper to the middle layers; then, press gently, with the circulate motion, into the deep layer (closer to the ribs) in the same spot. You should continue to repeat these steps as you inch your way from top to bottom in columns of the breast. Do the same exam technique in your underarm areas because breast tissue is also present there. Repeat on the other breast: Squeeze each nipple to make sure that blood discharge in not present. This exam should first be done lying down. Then, stand up and look in a mirror, clenching your fist into your hips and check for skin dimpling, nipple inversion, or skin bulging in your breasts. Finally, repeat the exam in the shower when the breasts are lathered with soap.

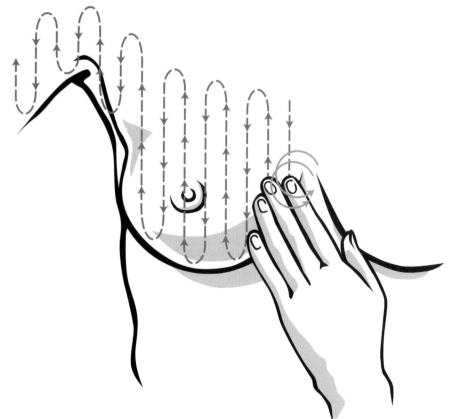

Use your index and middle finger to gently press in small circular motions.

Follow the path indicated by arrows in the diagram to the left. The path includes all of the breast and underarm area.

Clinical Breast Exam

Your clinician will repeat the same exam with you while you lie down as you did at home. Sometimes, the clinician will have you sit or stand for part of your breast exam.

Mammogram

If you have few risks for breast cancer, then early screening benefits you less. The older you are, the higher your risk of breast cancer and the greater the benefit of a mammogram every one to two years. Research on 10,000 women has shown that screening in your 30s or 40s for breast cancer can increase the number of false-positive mammograms, which then can result in increased fear, anxiety, and number of biopsies. Early screening would increase the life expectancy of only four women. This is why there is so much controversy as to when you should start your screening mammograms. Although four lives saved out of 10,000 lives may seem like a small statistical number, if it were your life that was saved by the early screening then it was absolutely worth screening early!

A mammogram is currently the most accurate and cost effective* test available to detect breast cancer, but it is not perfect. If you feel a lump, and your mammogram is negative, you may want a further test or biopsy performed. Breast tissue in your 30s and 40s can have more calcium deposits, be denser, and have more fibrous tissue making it more difficult to interpret your results.

It is not clear as to what age you can stop getting mammograms. Because your risk increases as you age, you may want to continue getting mammograms as long as you are in overall good health.

There are other tests available to detect breast cancer. These include magnetic resonance imaging (MRI), ultrasound, computed tomography (cat scan), and thermography (breast temperature used to detect breast cancer). There is also a computer analysis that can be done on your mammogram to confirm the radiologist's opinion.

If a mammogram or other screening test detects a lump, you may need to have further evaluation. This could include additional mammogram views, ultrasound,** or a biopsy. If you found a lump, and your mammogram was negative, you may still need a biopsy.

The biopsy can be done by a doctor using a needle that is inserted into the lump and fluid or cells are drawn out for further evaluation. Another biopsy technique is to surgically remove the lump, so it can then be looked at under a microscope. A radiologist may be asked to help locate your lump using three-dimensional (stereotactic) low dose x-ray. Your lump can be analyzed for estrogen and progesterone receptors. If your lump tests positive for estrogen receptors, you may have a better prognosis because of newer medicines that work at the receptor site. If your lump has positive estrogen and progesterone receptors, your prognosis may be even better. Knowing if you have estrogen and/or progesterone receptors will help you choose treatment options.

*Some states have Women's Health programs that will assist you in paying for a mammogram if your insurance doesn't cover it.
**Ultrasound helps to show if a lump is solid or fluid-filled.

Breast Lumps

Your breasts have many types of lumps. If you have lumpy breasts, sometimes doing a breast exam can be challenging; it can seem like you are feeling a bag full of marbles and trying to determine which one is the shooter. Normal anatomy of your breast includes fibrous tissue for support, milk glands and ducts that produce milk, and fatty tissue for insulation. The breast tissue starts on your chest wall and comes outward to form the breast. You also have "the tail of Spence" breast tissue that extends to your under arm. Your breast exams should include all of these areas.

There are several breast conditions that can cause a breast lump. These are benign or non-cancer conditions.

Benign Breast Lumps

Cyst: Fluid-filled sacs. They feel rubbery, smooth, tender, and mobile. Sometimes cysts need to be drained by your doctor if you continue to feel chronic discomfort.

Fibroadenoma: Made of fibrous and gland tissue. They feel smooth and rubbery, non-tender, and mobile. Can be surgically removed if they are getting larger or are bothersome.

Fibrocystic Breasts: Fibrous and cystic areas. The fibrous component will feel stringy or like a knotted cord. The cystic component will feel smooth, tender, and be a mobile discrete lump.

Fibrocystic breasts are sensitive to hormone changes and caffeine. Breast tenderness can be exaggerated around ovulation or menses hormone changes. Caffeine products like tea, coffee, chocolate, or medicines with caffeine can make your breasts more tender. Remember that "decaffeinated" really means **decreased caffeine, not caffeine-free**. To relieve the tenderness from fibrocystic breasts use comfortable bras, anti-inflammatories, warm moist heat, and decrease caffeine intake. Cancerous lumps are usually irregularly shaped, non-mobile, firm, and may be tender or non-tender. There are various cancerous breast lumps.

Cancerous Breast Lumps

In-situ Carcinoma: Located only in the breast duct. Seen more often in a younger patient. Early screening helps detect.

Ductal Carcinoma In situ: The most common type seen in patients in their 30s and 40s. Forms a localized palpable lump. Often has microcalcifications seen on mammogram. Can become invasive and aggressive if not treated. The lump can be surgically removed.

Lobular Carcinoma In situ: Occurs most often in premenopausal women. It does not have a palpable mass. It is found by mammogram. Patients often have had a history of atypical hyperplasia. Can be invasive.

Invasive Ductal and Lobular Tumors: Most invasive. Medullary and tubular types have a better prognosis.

Prognosis and Treatment

Prognosis and treatment depends on the type, size, and location of the tumor. If no lymph nodes are involved, then the prognosis is better. The smaller tumors may also have a better prognosis. Treatment choices range from various types of mastectomies and lymph node removal to breast conservative lumpectomy and radiation therapy. Conservative lumpectomy with radiation is not advised for invasive breast cancer due to a higher recurrence rate if used for treatment. Chemotherapy, when added to the initial therapy, seems to decrease recurrence rates for most all patients. If the tumor is estrogen-receptor positive, then giving tamoxifen for five years may help to decrease breast cancer recurrence rate. Tamoxifen is also being given to prevent breast cancer from ever occurring in women who are at high risk. Tamoxifen is not for everyone. It may increase blood clots and uterus cancer.

Also, Raloxifene (Evista) seems to reduce the risk of breast cancer in women who are postmenopausal. Evista and tamoxifen are selective estrogen receptor modulators (SERM). Evista is approved only to be given to postmenopausal women for osteoporosis prevention and treatment; Evista may increase blood clots. Several current studies being conducted (that should be completed in the next few years) will provide us with more information about other prevention treatment options.

Breast Health Highlights
(Breast screening suggestions)

	Age 30–39	Age 40–49	Age 50+
Self breast exams	Monthly	Monthly	Monthly
Clinical breast exams	Yearly	Yearly	Yearly
Mammograms	Screen if high risk	Every 1–2 years	Yearly

- See a physician for breast skin bulging, a new lump, dimpling, retracted nipple, bloody nipple discharge, or a lump that concerns you.
- See a physician for any lump that is new, irregularly shaped, non-mobile, tender or non-tender.
- Reassess your risks yearly, do self breast exams, clinical exams, and mammograms.
- Eighty percent of breast lumps are found by you doing your own self breast exam. Do a self exam monthly.
- For premenopausal self breast exam, do one week after your menses. For postmenopausal self breast exam, do first day of each month. If premenopausal, mammogram should be one week after your menses.
- If you feel a lump and the mammogram is negative, you may still need a biopsy.

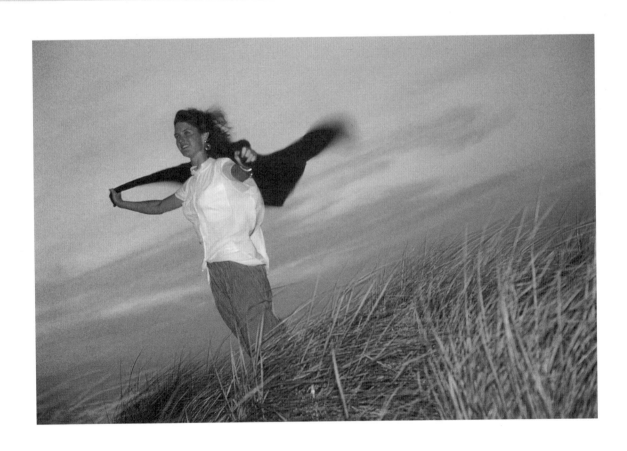

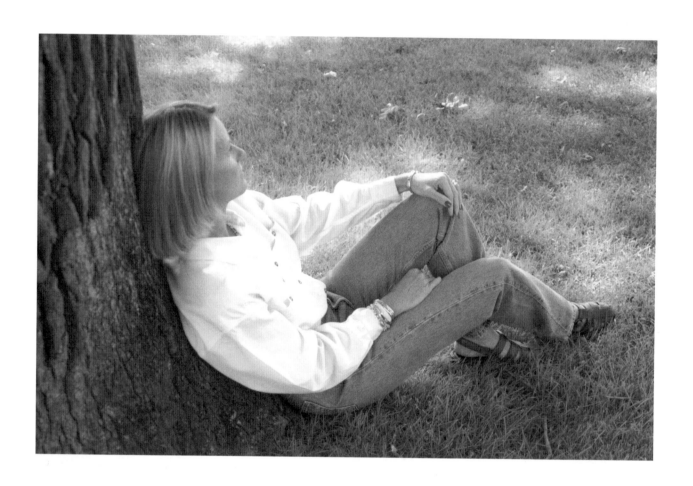

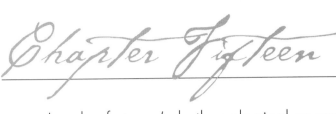

Levels of stress (whether physical or emotional) or diet changes can interfere with your hormone signals and cause your hormones to be imbalanced—therefore changing your sense of well-being.

Chapter 15: Your Hormones Up Close and Personal

How are your hormones made?

Your hormones are the key messengers from your brain that unlock a cascade of chemical reactions that allow your body to function effortlessly on autopilot all day and night. Your hormones regulate your body's functions in miraculous harmony to give you a sense of well-being and balance. Hormone messengers are made from protein or cholesterol; because these messengers are made from cholesterol, they belong to the family of steroid hormones.

Pregnenolone is the main steroid hormone, and is made from cholesterol. Pregnenolone then goes through a cascade of chemical reactions to create progesterone, estrogen, testosterone (yes, we have it too!), dehydroepiandrosterone (DHEA), cortisol, and aldosterone.

The harmony and balance of the above hormones' production is regulated by your brain and parts of your body. Hormone signals act as keys when inserted into organ tissue receptor locks. The hormone key unlocks the organ to do a specific thing like the FSH key unlocks your ovary to make estrogen.

Your body makes estrogen in three main forms. **Estrone** (E1) is the primary estrogen produced **after** menopause. Estrone is made from your adipose (fat) tissue (see—we need that fat for something!). **Estradiol** (E2) is the most potent estrogen; it is produced by your ovaries, and it makes up to 10–20 percent of your total estrogen. Estradiol is the primary estrogen produced **before** menopause. Estrone (E1) and Estradiol (E2) can be converted by your body to make **Estriol** (E3); this hormone makes up 60–90 percent of your total estrogen. The levels of Estrone, Estradiol, and Estriol vary depending on where you're at in your life cycle, menstrual years, perimenopause, or menopause.

Levels of stress, whether physical or emotional, or diet changes can interfere with your hormone signals and cause your hormones to be unbalanced—therefore changing your sense of well-being.

Hormones: Up Close and Personal

Estrogen
Estrogen helps to regulate the health of your uterus, ovaries, breast, skin, and brain. Estrogen is what makes you look feminine by regulating your distribution of fat to your breasts and hips. Estrogen helps maintain calcium for strong bones and maintains vagina moisture.

Progesterone
Progesterone helps shed the uterus lining by a menses if an egg was not fertilized. It helps protect against uterus cancer by putting on the brakes if there is too much estrogen present in your uterus. Progesterone also acts as a natural water pill. It helps build bone, maintain glucose (sugar) usage, maintain libido, and improve restorative sleep.

Androgens
Androgens include dehydroepiandrosterone (DHEA) and testosterone. The DHEA hormone may help with energy, mood, and mental function. Testosterone helps maintain muscle, bone, skin, hair, and libido.

Cortisol
Cortisol is a glucocorticoid made by the adrenal glands. Cortisol helps you handle stress, exercise, and regulate your immune system against inflammation and infection. Cortisol helps maintain your brain's fuel, which is blood sugar (glucose). Excessive stress (emotional or physical), extreme dieting (eliminating carbs or proteins) can cause your adrenal gland to go into overdrive and become exhausted to the point of causing a decline in cortisol production. Cortisol production can leave you with low blood sugar, causing mental and physical fatigue.

As you can see, hormones provide you with a sense of harmony, balance, and well-being. When your hormones are no longer working, this creates disharmony and imbalance. When you are in perimenopause (the nine years prior to your last period) or menopause (your last period was six months ago) your hormone levels change and can cause symptoms. Are you experiencing perimenopause or menopause symptoms? Take a look at the list of symptoms that can occur when your estrogen, progesterone, DHEA, testosterone, or cortisol levels change.

Perimenopause and Menopause Symptoms:*

Hot flashes	Night sweats	Vaginal dryness
Heart palpitations	Depression	Anxiety
Urinary incontinence	Fatigue	Bone loss
Sleep disturbances	Memory loss	Foggy thinking
Moodiness/Irritability	Food cravings	Water retention
Weight changes	Decreased sex drive	Irregular menses

What do Hormones do?
Hormones regulate your body functions; it all starts automatically in your brain. Everything from your body temperature, insulin production, reproductive cycle, to your sense of well-being, is regulated by hormones. Your hypothalamus and pituitary gland secrete hormones to your thyroid, pancreas, adrenal glands, and ovaries. Some of these hormone messengers (follicle stimulating hormone (FSH) and luteinizing hormone (LH)) tell the ovaries how much estrogen and progesterone to make for you. There is a "negative" feedback to your brain to stop production of that hormone when your body has made enough of a particular hormone for the time being.

*Always get a thyroid stimulating hormone level (TSH) drawn to eliminate thyroid imbalance as a cause for your symptoms.

By the time of menopause, your ovaries have grown smaller and aren't functioning like they used to when you were younger. Before menopause, if your egg didn't get fertilized, your body increased its hormone progesterone to shed the prepared uterus lining (womb) in the form of a menses.

At menopause, your ovaries aren't functioning to release that egg, so your hormone messengers send back a message to your brain that your ovaries aren't "listening" and aren't releasing an egg. Your brain responds to this received message that your ovaries aren't "listening" and sends an even "bigger" message of FSH to scream at the ovaries to do what they are told to do and release the egg. That is why one of the ways to check to see if you are in menopause is to have your doctor get a FSH level. FSH levels elevated higher than 30, no menses for six months, and menopause symptoms can help you confirm that you are in menopause.

Hormone Testing

Let's face it, some days you could check "yes" to most of the symptoms listed for perimenopause or menopause. If your symptoms are interfering with your life, you may choose to discuss testing and/or treatment options with your doctor. Hormone level testing is not necessary to establish that you are in perimenopause. You do not have to have hormone levels tested or have a follicle stimulating hormone (FSH) level drawn to confirm menopause. Having vaginal dryness, hot flashes, night sweats, and having had no menses for over six months can be enough to confirm menopause. Menopause is usually around 51 years of age, but it can happen earlier. If you are experiencing symptoms of menopause in your 30s or 40s, you may want testing done to confirm that your symptoms are actually being caused by menopause (versus something like a thyroid disorder).

If you want some form of an official test of menopause, you can get a serum/blood level of FHS. Along with symptoms, an FSH>30 mg/dl can help to confirm menopause.

There are other tests are available that can show your other hormone levels. These tests can be done by serum or saliva. Some feel that saliva testing is the only way to get an accurate progesterone level that is "bioavailable," or free (not bound up at a work site, but is free for your body to use where needed in the blood stream). Serum (blood) levels of hormones are tested for you at a doctor's office. Saliva testing* can be done at home and then mailed by you to a testing facility. It is best to do hormone testing on day 21 of your cycle, or when off of estrogen or progesterone at least seven days.

*Saliva test kits are available from natural compounding pharmacies, special labs, and some clinics.

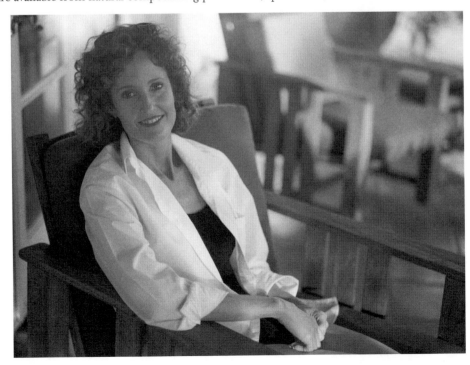

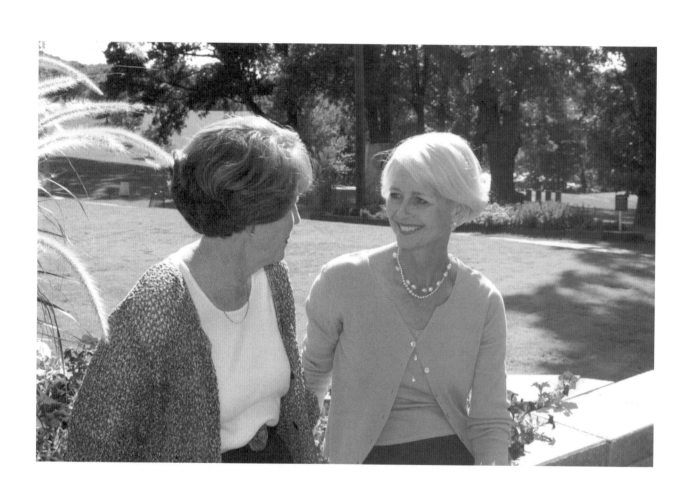

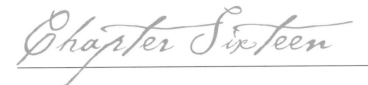

Chapter Sixteen

Of course, you are almost ready with your final decision—just in time to be swayed 180 degrees to a different choice after the media releases a health tip about HRT from a newer study that now makes you second guess and rethink your original decision.

Chapter 16: Hormone Replacement Therapy What is the Right Choice for You?

As I walked into the exam room, I could feel the heavy tension in the air. There sat my patient's husband, Rick, in the corner visitor chair; if body language speaks to an observer, his body was screaming. His arms were tightly folded across his chest. He wore a frown, and scrunched eyelids revealed dark, angry eyes flashing my way as I entered into the room. My patient, his wife Mary, sat slumped on the exam table with tearful eyes cast down toward the floor. She clutched a tear-soaked tissue. Her facial expression looked hopeless and helpless. Rick's booming words echoed off the small exam room wall as I tried to soak in the picture before me in order to assess the situation. "All she does is cry, and when she is not crying she acts like she is going to." His frustrated tone continued, "She is having so many hot flashes and mood swings she can't even function. We can't do anything together like we used to be able to." His voice then roared with a clutched fist waving in the air with desperation. "Fix her! I want my wife back!" In other words he wanted his and her life back as it was before the symptoms-of-decreased-estrogen-because-of-menopause happened.

I confirmed that Mary was, indeed, in menopause and that this was causing her symptoms. During the next visit, we talked about her risks and benefits for her going on a short-term customized hormone replacement therapy plan. For her, it was a good decision. Within months Mary returned for an exam—smiling again and saying she was having fewer hot flashes, less tearfulness, and fewer mood swings, and had a better sense of well-being.

Whether or not to take HRT seems to be a question looming in front of all of us in our 40s and early 50s. The decision to take HRT seems overwhelming by the time you plunge through all the confusing—and often contradictory—information; you struggle with assessing the risks and benefits, as well as becoming better informed about the different types and doses and methods of taking hormone replacement therapy. This monumental decision seems almost as life-defining and as life-changing as choosing a partner or the career to which you are going to give your energy and talents. The decision, whether or not to take HRT seems like such a permanent decision—that once you make it, you can't turn back or change your mind. As we will discuss later, this is not the case. First you take into consideration what your mother did (didn't talk about it—silent passage, or doesn't remember the details), what Aunt Ruth did (just got through it), or your friends and their hormone replacement therapy "war stories." And then when you find enough time to go through all the TV, magazine, and radio information, you then feel you finally have enough information to make a decision. Of course, you are almost ready with your final decision—just in time to be swayed 180 degrees to a different choice after the media releases a health tip about HRT from a newer study that now makes you second guess and rethink your original decision! No wonder we start to look gray and wrinkled in our 40s!

It can be stressful to try and make the "right" decision about whether or not to take HRT, and then having to try and live with the consequences of your decision "forever." Why can't someone just print, in one paragraph, what is the best and right decision for you?

The decision of whether or not to take HRT should not be this painstakingly difficult. Do you have to take hormone replacement therapy? Simply put—no. The FDA has approved three reasons to take HRT: 1) To treat hot flashes 2) For atrophic vaginitis (dry, painful vagina or vulvar area) 3) To prevent osteoporosis. Hot flashes, atrophic (aging cells) vaginitis, and osteoporosis are signs and symptoms of decreased estrogen in your body. Studies have proven that estrogen replacement therapy can treat or prevent these signs and symptoms. What makes the decision of whether or not to take hormone replacement therapy more challenging is all of the benefits or risks being discussed about estrogen.

A recent study showed that taking 0.625 mg of conjugated equine estrogen plus 2.5 mg medroxyprogesterone slightly increased the number of invasive breast cancers, blood clots, heart attacks, and strokes compared to women who were not taking this estrogen and progestin combination. This study also shows the benefit of fewer cases of colon cancer and hip fractures. **Overall, it is felt that the risks of taking long-term estrogen and progestin combinations outweigh the benefits for most women.**

Despite the FDA approved reasons to take estrogen, this recent study shows that most women should first choose options other than taking estrogen to treat hot flashes, atrophic vaginitis, or to prevent osteoporosis.

Options, other than estrogen, exist for the treatment of hot flashes, vaginal dryness or atrophy, and osteoporosis. Short-term usage of oral estrogen does work well for disabling hot flashes if other options have not helped and if you do not have risk factors for taking it. For vaginal dryness, use lubrication or intravaginal estrogen in the form of a dissolving tablet or ring. Intravaginal estrogen does not go through your liver like oral estrogen does. For the prevention of osteoporosis, do daily exercises, light weight toning, eat calcium-rich foods, or take a calcium supplement. If you need treatment or prevention, the bisphonate products (Fosomax, Actonel) work well. For some women with hot flashes, foods with phytoestrogens and/or serotonin reuptake inhibitor medicines seem to help relieve their symptoms.

Hormone replacement therapy is not for everyone, and there are a few of you for whom it is absolutely contraindicated in. If you do choose to take hormone replacement therapy, "one size" doesn't fit everyone, and you should have your own personalized, short-term usage plan for hormone replacement therapy consultation with your physician. A decision of type, dose, strength, length of time to take, and method does not have to be made for a lifetime—never to be changed or altered again.

Matter of fact, a more reasonable approach if you choose to take HRT is to make a short-term plan that will hopefully give you lifelong benefits. This customized hormone replacement therapy plan should be reevaluated every year by you and your physician based on your current symptoms and healthcare needs. By reevaluating every year, you will keep your hormone replacement therapy plan appropriate to your current healthcare needs, and you will stay current with the newest medical research.

Tips for HRT:

- Using short-term hormone replacement therapy is a personal choice based on your signs, symptoms, lifestyle, and risk factors for disease.
- Hormone replacement therapy is not for everyone. There may be absolute contraindications for your taking HRT that would cause you greater risk than benefit. See your doctor.
- Reassess your HRT plan and decision every year; this will enable you to update your plan and to remain current with the newest medical research.
- Regardless of your decision of whether or not to take short-term HRT, invest in yourself: eat sensible, healthy meals that include fruits and vegetables every day, exercise regularly, stop smoking, get a routine pap smear, mammogram, and physical exams, drink 64 ounces of water daily, stop consuming caffeine, and become fit and fabulous.

Question and Answer

Question #1: Do I have to take hormone replacement therapy?

Answer: No. Whether to take HRT or not is your own personal decision. For most women, a long-term estrogen and progestin combination may have more risks than benefits. If you have disabling hot flashes that are resistant to any other treatment, then a short-term estrogen/progestin combination may be of benefit to you.

Question #2: Will you please explain the recent media release about the risks and benefits of hormone replacement therapy?

Answer: In an attempt to study the risks and benefits of estrogen and progestin combination therapy, the Women's Health Initiative (WHI) enrolled 16,608 postmenopausal women, with intake uteri, into a trial study between 1993 and 1998. In the study, 8,506 women received an estrogen and progestin combination (0.625 mg conjugated equine estrogen plus 2.5 mg medroxyprogesterone acetate) and 8,102 women received a placebo. The study was scheduled to be completed in March 2005. The WHI stopped the study of the estrogen and progestin combination therapy on May 2002, after 5.2 years, when it became apparent that the health risks exceeded the benefits.

The WHI study showed that the estrogen and progestin combination increased risk of getting coronary heart disease, stroke, pulmonary embolus (blood clot in the lung), and invasive breast cancer. The combination hormone therapy decreased your risk of colorectal cancer and hip fracture.

If the study was expanded to 10,000 women, it would mean that there would be seven more cases of heart disease, eight more strokes, eight more pulmonary emboli, and eight more invasive cancers of the breast; however, this would also mean six fewer cancers of the colorectal area and five fewer hip fractures. In other words, there would be 20 more health events that would happen to 10,000 women than if they had not taken the estrogen and progestin combination. Overall, the risks of taking a long-term estrogen and progestin combination outweigh the benefits and should not be taken by most women, except for the short-term treatment of hot flashes.

The study showed that the estrogen and progestin combination should not be used for the prevention of coronary heart disease. Based on the WHI study, HRT will not be a first choice therapy for osteoporosis prevention or treatment. There have been no large studies on the risks, benefits, or safety of natural or bioidentical estrogen or progesterone combinations. It has not been studied to see if other combinations, types, or doses of estrogen, progesterone, or progestin, or patches, creams, etc., are any safer. It is currently thought that a women without a uterus taking only estrogen can continue her treatment. Also, perimenopausal women taking birth control pills to control symptoms can continue if they do not smoke and are otherwise healthy without diabetes, lupus, high blood pressure, or heart disease.

Question #3: Based on the WHI study, should I stop my hormone replacement therapy?

Answer: First, you must look at your personal risks and benefits. If the only reason you have been taking HRT is to prevent heart disease, then you need to talk to your doctor about stopping HRT. If you are at an increased risk for heart disease, stroke, pulmonary embolus, or breast cancer, and you are at a low risk for colorectal cancer and hip fracture, you may need to consider other options. If you are having disabling hot flashes resistent to other treatment, and have no risks for taking HRT, then short-term estrogen treatment may be of a benefit to you.

Remember that heart disease, stroke, pulmonary embolus, breast cancer, colorectal cancer, and hip fractures can occur even if you do not have any family history or risk factors for them. If HRT is stopped, you may have bone density loss without the estrogen. Talk to your doctor about getting a bone density screen.

Question #4: What is the best way to stop HRT?

Answer: First of all, please do not stop your HRT without discussing the risks and benefits with your doctor. No studies show the best way to stop HRT. Abrupt stopping or tapering off of HRT are the two choices for stopping HRT. You may experience spotting or hot flashes when hormones are stopped.

Question #5: Why should I take HRT?

Answer: The FDA has approved three reasons to take HRT: for hot flashes (vasomotor symptoms), vaginal or vulvar dryness (or aging tissue), or to prevent osteoporosis. Based on the WHI study, HRT will not be the first choice therapy for osteoporosis prevention or treatment; also, you should first choose other options to treat hot flashes or vaginal dryness. Vaginal dryness that is resistant to with other treatment can be treated (in most women) with vaginal estrogen.

If you do choose to use HRT to treat hot flashes, vaginal dryness, and/or to prevent osteoporosis, you should use it **only short-term** and reevaluate your decision yearly. If you can not function because of your hot flashes, vaginal dryness, or you have marked osteoporosis, then taking short-term HRT may be a choice for you if the benefits outweigh the risks of hormone replacement therapy.

Question #6: When should an estrogen and progestin combination not be used?

Answer: Estrogen and progestin should not be used with the following: pregnancy, breast cancer, undiagnosed vaginal bleeding, disorders with blood clots, history of stroke, or liver disease.

Question #7: What are alternatives of taking HRT for menopausal symptoms and preventing heart disease and osteoporosis?

Answer: See chart on following pages

Symptoms/Condition	Alternative	Amount	Comments
Hot flashes and night sweats (raised body temp, artery dilatation, sweating leads to moodiness, stress, insomnia)	Soy (phytoestrogen)* Exercise	25–60 grams a day 30 minutes daily	25 grams is a safe amount
	Progesterone cream	Varies by type	May alter lipid levels, increase fatigue
	Diet	Increase fruits and veggies	
	Black cohosh	Varies	Use for less than 6 months, RemiFemin Menopause is similar to German brand
	Red clover	Varies	Pill contains extracted plant estrogens that are made synthetic (its market name is Promensil)
	Effexor SR	37.5–75 mg per day	(antidepressant) less hot flashes
	Paxil	20 mg per day	(antidepressant) less hot flashes
	Lifestyle	Avoid alcohol, caffeine, pop	can cause insomnia and decrease bone density
	No studies have found other herbal or homeopathic treatments to control hot flashes other than these listed**		
Heart disease prevention (see heart chapter for more details)	Lifestyle	Maintain a healthy weight, keep blood pressure 130/85 or less, maintain blood sugar at 110 mg/dl, don't smoke, control cholesterol, LDL triglycerides, decrease stress, exercise	Eat a balanced variety of foods, include food that have fish oil, omega-3 like deep ocean fish, tuna, salmon, (see nutrition and vitamin chapters)
	Soy	25 grams a day	Soy helps to lower cholesterol and LDL
	Multivitamins	One tablet	Should include vitamins A, B, C, and E, folic acid
	Be happy		Happiness is a habit, think 3 positive thoughts each morning when you wake up
	Lipid-lowering medicine	Depends on meds	May need if lifestyle changes do not result in successfully lowering lipids
	Aspirin	81 mg per day	If okayed by doctor

*Soy is not as effective on hot flashes if on Tamoxifen. It is not known whether or not you need to protect the uterus from cancer with progesterone when using soy products.

**Natural, or bioidentical products may have the same risks as synthetic.

© 2002 Dr. Robin Hartley

Chart continued on following page

Symptoms/Condition	Alternative	Amount	Comments
Bone loss (see osteoporosis chart)	Soy*	25–60 g per day	May increase spine density, 25 g is safe
	Exercise	Walk 30 minutes daily, free weights or resistance machines alternating days	
	Calcium	1,200 mg per day (1,500mg per day if postmenopausal)	Eat calcium rich foods, consider supplements if needed (see osteoporosis chapter)
	Magnesium	One multivitamin plus fruits, veggies, dairy, meat	If deficient will decrease bone density, helps to suppress your parathyroid hormone so more calcium is retained

*If at an increased risk for fracture or osteoporosis, then you may need Flosomax, Actonel, or Evista for prevention.

Vaginal Dryness	Lubricants		Petrol jelly, vegetable shortening is not as drying as jelly
	Intravaginal estrogen	Cream, tablet, or ring	Most prefer tablet or ring

Question #8: Can you summarize estrogen?
Answer: See chart below*

FDA Approved Reasons to Take	Increases Risk of	Contraindicated If you have...	Side Effects	Benefits
Hot flashes night sweats, vaginal dryness, prevent osteoporosis**	Heart disease, breast cancer, stroke, blood clots, gallstones, endometrial cancer (if not taking progesterone)	Breast cancer, uterine cancer, stroke, blood clots, unexplained, uterine bleeding, pregnancy, nursing, or active liver disease	Breast tenderness, bloating, weight gain	Fewer cases of colon cancer or hip fractures, reduction of instances of hot flashes, night sweats, vaginal dryness, prevent osteoporosis

*Use estrogen for less than five years to decrease risk of breast cancer. Once HRT is stopped, it takes five years to return to pre-estrogen risk level. Increased risk of heart attack, stroke, and blood clots happen as early as the first few years of estrogen/progestin usage. If you decide to continue on short-term HRT, get yearly mammograms and make healthy lifestyle choices to decrease your risk of heart disease or osteoporosis and reevaluate your decision yearly. Evaluate, with your doctor, the risks and benefits of taking short-term HRT. Get a physical, pap, pelvic, colon study, mammogram, and bone density test. Lab may include complete cholesterol levels. Look at your family, personal, and social/lifestyle history to determine your risk for heart disease, breast cancer, and osteoporosis (see related chapters for risk profiles.)

**Based on the WHI study, estrogen may not be the first choice therapy for osteoporosis prevention or treatment.

Question #9: What can I do about night sweats?

Answer: Hot flashes and night sweats may be caused by your body raising its core temperature and your arteries dilating. These changes cause you to feel warm. Hot flashes and night sweats are not harmful, but they can cause a cascade effect on your life. The feeling of being hot and then cold (covers on/covers off during the night), causes sleep disturbances that leave you feeling fatigued and irritable. This can then cause personal disharmony with your partner, family, friends, and co-workers. Instead of feeling refreshed and restored in the morning, you feel fatigued.

Tips for Hot Flashes and Night Sweats:

- Dress in layers: Remove or add clothing to keep you comfortable and to better control your climate.
- Exercise: Helps to regulate body temperature
- Diet: Eat a healthy, balanced diet. Avoid spicy, hot foods, nicotine, alcohol, caffeine (and other stimulants like decongestants).
- Bedtime: Wear a cotton nightgown or pajamas. Use cotton sheets, blankets, bed spreads (satin, down, polyester, and flannel reflect your body heat back to you). Take a warm bath to relax before bed. Keep the bedroom for sleep or intimacy—not for work or entertainment. Keep it dark— light can cause arousal. Try to stay on schedule with the same bedtime and wake up at the same time most days.
- Relax: Use relaxation techniques like controlled breathing, visualization, biofeedback, and massage.

Question #10: What are the possible side effects of HRT?

Answer: Common side effects of HRT include breast tenderness, irregular menses, and bloating. Absolute contraindications for taking HRT are undiagnosed urine bleeding, severe liver disease, breast feeding, or pregnancy. Also, you should let your doctor know about all prescriptions and over-the-counter products you are taking. Even Tylenol or garlic pills may have potential side effects or drug interactions with products.

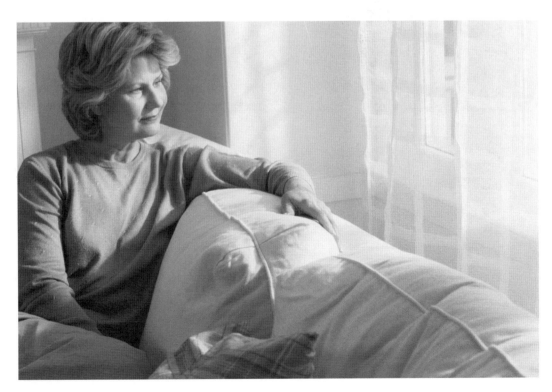

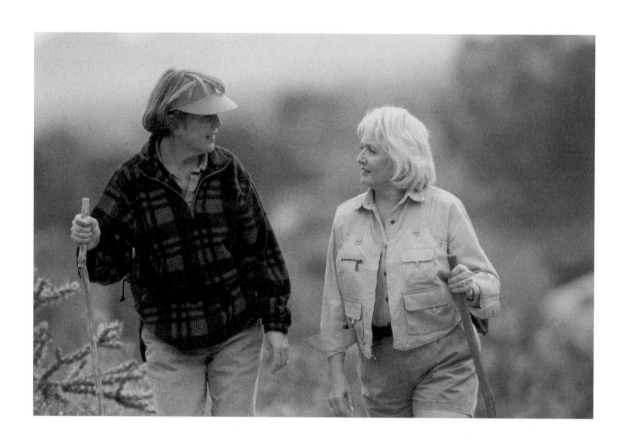

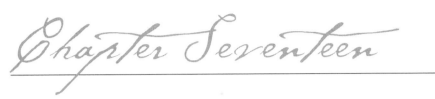

Chapter Seventeen

It could be made in a lab and still be called "natural," as long as it is bioidentically the same as the product made by your body.

Chapter 17: Hormone Replacement Therapy Natural vs. Synthetic

Lynn knew that she was opposed to taking hormone replacement therapy. She had heard "war stories" of the side effects that HRT could cause—like irregular bleeding, breast tenderness, and weight gain. Lynn also had a fear of breast cancer because her grandmother had breast cancer.

Until now, Lynn had felt she was getting along just fine with her menopausal symptoms. However, recently she had begun to feel that her hot flashes and moodiness were consuming her life. During the night, Lynn would have intense hot flashes that caused her to kick the covers off and pull the covers back on all night long. That left her feeling tired and irritable during the day, and we all know that if Mom is in a bad mood, no one in the family can be in a good mood.

Lynn knew several of her friends who had tried products like soy, black cohosh, primrose, and over-the-counter progesterone cream. Some of her friends seemed to be having good luck with these natural products relieving their menopausal symptoms. After all, natural is better than synthetic, isn't it?

After her father had a hip fracture from a fall, Lynn decided to get a bone density test performed. The bone density test showed Lynn had normal bone density.

As a result of suffering from intense hot flashes, she decided it was time to see her doctor. With her doctor, Lynn was able to rationalize her fears, emotions, and preconceived opinion of hormone replacement therapy. After looking at her personal risks and benefits for short-term hormone replacement therapy, Lynn felt the benefits outweighed the risks. Lynn chose to take a synthetic HRT on a short-term basis to help control her hot flashes.

Lynn returned for a follow-up visit and was thrilled to say that she was "back on top" of things and in better control of her life. Her hot flashes were completely gone and she felt more energized with improved sleep. Taking short-term HRT to control disabling hot flashes was the right decision for her.

Hormone Replacement Therapy

So how do you decide whether natural or synthetic is right for you? For most of your life, you have been taught that if something is natural it is more pure, wholesome, or healthier for you. Fresh air, pure spring water, and homegrown vegetables and fruits are examples of things that are good for you. And you may have thought that man-made would not be as good for you "with all those chemicals." If you stop and think about it, what is natural isn't always safe and wholesome (i.e. marijuana, tobacco) and what is man-made isn't always bad (i.e. insulin, IV fluid).

It may come as no surprise to you to learn that a hormone replacement therapy product is called "natural" if it has the same chemical structure (bioidentical) as the product your body makes. However, it may surprise you to learn that a **natural** product can be made from a plant, animal, or be **chemically made** or modified. Just because it says it is natural doesn't necessarily mean that it is from nature. It could be made in a lab and be called "natural," as long as it is bioidentically the same as the product made by your body. Hormone replacement therapy that is called "**synthetic**" or "man-made" can be chemically made or modified, or **plant or animal derived**! A synthetic or man-made product could have originally come from a plant or animal source, but can not be called natural if it is not bioidentical to the product made by your body.

Synthetic HRT Sources Available for Estrogen or Progesterone	
Sources of Estrogen	**Brand Name**
Pregnant mare's urine	Premarin
Mexican yam	Ogen, Ortho-est, Estinyl, Estraderm, Vivelle, Estring
Soy	Menest, Climara, Femhrt
Soy and yam	Cenestin, Estratab, Estrace, Combipatch
Pregnant mare's urine and synthetic progesterone (medroxyprogesterone acetate)	PremPro, Premphase
Soy or yam + synthetic	EstraTest, OrthoPrefest
Synthetic	Alora, FemPatch, Activella,
Progesterone	
Mexican yam	Prometrium, Crinone
Synthetic	Provera, Cycrin

Natural Hormone Replacement Therapy

Natural hormone replacement therapy provides you with an alternative choice to the standard synthetic hormone replacement therapy. Synthetic (man-made) HRT has to go through testing to meet FDA approval in order to be marketed and sold based on efficacy and safety. The synthetic product can be patented and has to go through quality control standards that guarantee that each product contains the exact ingredients and proportions as listed on the label. Because a patented product can generate more research dollars from its profits, all of the current data and research on HRT has been done on synthetic HRT.

Natural HRT can receive a "process patent" which gives credit for how the product was made. The FDA currently does not regulate the quality of natural HRT, herbs, or vitamin products. Natural compounding pharmacies and pharmacists are licensed and inspected by their individual state pharmacy board. Most of the natural products are under the good manufacturing procedures code. Natural HRT can not be patented because natural HRT lack the large profits that patented HRT have to allow research data; no significant studies have been conducted to establish natural HRT efficacy or safety. With natural HRT, the natural compounding pharmacist has the ability to make customized products for you. The choices include pills, capsules, gels, troches (lozenges), oral drops, creams, or injections. Compounding pharmacists can leave out preservatives, colors, or chemicals that can cause you allergies or sensitivities; they can also add flavors or make specialized products for you.

Note: Over-the-counter natural hormones such as progesterone are from wild yam—but beware! The label must say "contains progesterone" because your body doesn't have the enzyme necessary to convert wild yam to progesterone.

How do human estrogen, synthetic estrogen, and natural estrogen compare?*

Human Estrogen	Synthetic (man-made) Premarin	Natural Compounded Triple Estrogen
Estrone 10–20%	Estrone 75–80%	Estrone 10%
Estradiol 10–20%	Estradiol 5–19%	Estradiol 20%
Estriol 60–80%	Equilin 6–15% (Estrogen from pregnant mares urine)	Estriol 70%

Natural HRT comes from the wild yam (*Diajcorea composita*). The wild yam is converted in a lab to "natural" or bioidentical estrogen, progesterone, or testosterone. When this conversion is completed, these hormones look like (are bioidentical) to the human hormone, so they are called "natural." There are several types of synthetic estrogen that also come from yam or soy sources.

Why can't you just sit down and eat a bowl of wild yams? Because you do not have the necessary enzymes in your body that can convert wild yam to a hormone.

Because natural HRT is not patented or made by large pharmacy companies, there are no brand names for the products. The natural compounding pharmacy is able to custom-make your natural product from hundreds of combinations of estrogen, progesterone, and testosterone. The most common products are triple estrogen (estrone/estradiol/estriol) or bi-estrogen (estradiol/estriol).

Synthetic hormone replacement therapy

Premarin is the most commonly used HRT. Synthetic HRT has been FDA approved to help stop hot flashes, vaginal dryness, and prevent osteoporosis.** Premarin is conjugated equine estrogen that blends pregnant mare's urine with other estrogens made from the Mexican yam.

Natural progesterone*** is a hormone manufactured from the Mexican yam. The earlier-made oral progesterones were poorly absorbed by the body, so synthetic progesterone was made. The most common synthetic progesterone is Provera (medroxyprogesterone acetate—MPA.)

The natural oral progesterone (OMP) absorption was later improved by making it micronized (making it tiny with more surface area). The most commonly used natural progesterone is Prometrium.

Hormone replacement therapy, whether it is natural or synthetic, is not for everyone. One-size-fits-all does not apply here. Recent data shows that long-term use of an estrogen and progestin combination therapy may slightly increase risks of breast cancer, stroke, blood clots, and heart attacks. However, it still is protective against hip fractures and colorectal cancer. The increased risks of taking HRT long term may outweigh the benefits. You will need to look at your own risks versus the benefits in order to decide if your should take short-term HRT. No current studies prove that natural HRT is safer than synthetic HRT. Natural HRT has not been FDA approved to treat or prevent hot flashes, vaginal dryness, or osteoporosis. If you are taking HRT because you have had a hysterectomy, you may need to continue taking estrogen only until age 50 to protect your bones. If continued protection is needed for your bones, so you may want to consider other options such as Fosomax, Actonel, or Evista (they are FDA approved for osteoporosis); taking 1,200–1,500 mg calcium with vitamin D, doing resistance exercises with weights or machines, doing weight-bearing exercises, and eating calcium-rich foods and soy products are natural options for continued bone protection.

For hot flashes, black cohosh and soy products help some women. Antidepressants Effexor (37.5–75 mg) or Paxil (20 mg) can also help with hot flashes.

For vaginal dryness, topical estrogen creams, tablets, or rings restore moisture without being as absorbed as an oral estrogen tablet. Lubricants also work to restore moisture to the vagina.

---

*Adapted from Dr. Jean Lorentzen, D.O.'s "Perspective of Hormone Replacement Therapy."
**Based on a recent study, estrogen may not be your first choice to prevent or treat osteoporosis.
***Progesterone should always be given to you when taking estrogen if you have a uterus. This protects you from uterine cancer. OMP and MPA seem equal in protecting the uterus. Progesterone creams and gels may not protect the uterus. Micronized progesterone is prepared in peanut oil; so, if you have a peanut allergy, you may need an oil-based micronized progesterone.

Question and Answer

Question #1: What about my diet?

Answer: You can eat phytoestrogens (plant estrogens) that act like estrogens, and may help relieve your symptoms of hot flashes and may protect your bones. The FDA has recommended 25 grams a day of soy protein food for heart protection. Phytoestrogens are considered a dietary supplement and are therefore not regulated. There are three types of phytoestrogens: isoflavones, lignans, and coumestans. The most common isoflavone is the soy bean. Soy products include curd (tofu), cake (tempeh), and paste (miso). Soy is also a source of calcium. The best source of soy is natural, organically-grown food products versus synthetic pill supplements. Good food sources for soy are soy milk, tofu, miso, or tempeh products. Other sources include flax seed, wheat, oat, rice, bean, legumes, broccoli, carrots, sweat potatoes, garlic, strawberries, and peas.

Question #2: What about the other over-the-counter products advertised to treat menopause symptoms?

Answer: There are many products being tried for relief of menopausal symptoms. Some of these products include dehydroepiandrosterone (DHEA), red clover, evening primrose oil, dong quai, kava-kava, clonidine, vitamin E, and Bellergal. These products have not been extensively studied for their menopausal symptom benefit. They can have side effects and may have serious drug interactions with other products that you consume. Discuss your options with your doctor before trying any product.

Question #3: How do I know when to start short-term HRT?

Answer: There is not one clear answer. Most of the time, it is your increasing menopausal symptoms that will tell you to see your doctor for HRT or other options. You and your doctor can review your symptoms, personal and family history review the risks versus benefits of short-term HRT, and consider drawing a follicle stimulating hormone (FSH) level. An FSH is not always accurate to diagnose menopause because it can fluctuate during the month. However, an FSH level (if greater than 30) can sometimes help to clarify whether or not you are in menopause. After starting HRT, estradiol levels can be drawn to determine if the estrogen dose you are taking is effective.

Question #4: Which form of HRT (oral , patch, or cream) is right for me?

Answer: The oral form is the form on which most of the current research has been done. The oral form goes through your intestine and your liver. Oral estrogen can affect your lipids (increase HDL and triglycerides, and decrease LDL and cholesterol), sex hormone binding globulin, clotting factors, and insulin-like growth factor. The transdermal patch is a better option for women who have had increased blood pressure with estrogen, gall bladder stones, history of venous thrombosis, or diabetes because the estrogen patch doesn't affect the liver the same way oral estrogen does. Progesterone cream absorption—and therefore effectiveness—may depend on how thin your skin is, where you apply it, how much you apply, how consistently you apply it, and what clothes you wear.

Question #5: Should I take cyclic or continuous HRT?

Answer: With either, you can expect some degree of irregular bleeding that could last up to one year. Estrogen and progesterone given continuously have the least amount of irregular bleeding. And it has been shown that an ethinyl estrogen and norethindrone acetate combination may be very effective at stopping the bleeding in the shortest amount of time. If you have bleeding with continuous estrogen and progestin, sometimes going to a different dose will stop the bleeding.

Question #6: When should I stop taking HRT?

Answer: First you need to reassess your HRT benefits each year. You need to know your risks and benefits and have no contraindications for taking short-term HRT. If you are not sure of any benefit you are getting, or have been taking HRT for heart disease prevention, then you need to consider other options. The risks of long-term HRT include increased stroke, heart attack, and breast cancer; these risks may outweigh your benefits of decreased colorectal cancer and hip fracture.

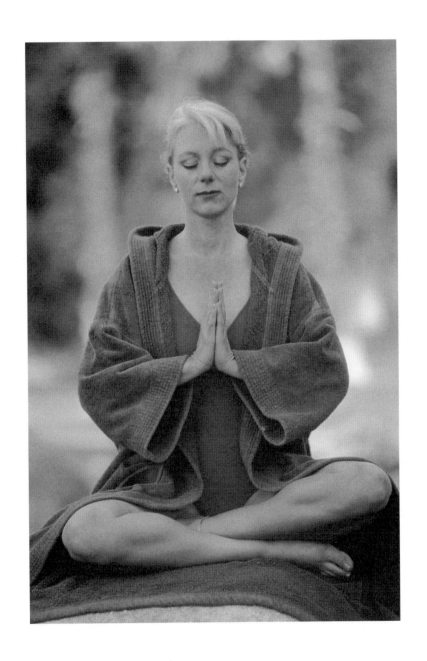

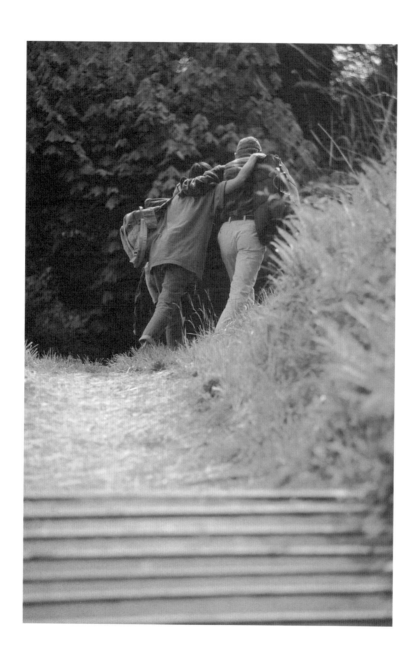

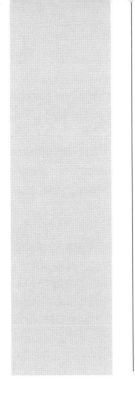

Chapter Eighteen

You may also have symptoms that are not typical; these symptoms include shortness of breath (with walking, exercise, or even at rest), chest heaviness, shoulder pain, or unexplained, persistent dizziness.

Chapter 18: Your Heart
Your Surprising Chance for Disease

You have a 1 in 4 chance of getting coronary artery disease (CAD) in your lifetime. And if you get coronary artery disease, you have a 1 in 2 (50 percent) chance that the CAD will kill you. In other words, look to the person on your left, on your right, and in front of you, and know that one of you will die of CAD.

This is very sobering when you consider that you have been spending a lot of time worrying about your chances of getting breast cancer and not about your chances of getting heart disease. It is statistically more likely that it will be your coronary arteries that kill you.

Your chance for getting breast cancer, if you live into your 90s, is 1 in 8. Out of the 25 people that will get breast cancer, one will die from it. Again, your chance for getting coronary artery disease is 1 in 4. Out of the four people that will get CAD, two will die from it! These are not good odds.*

Are you reading this and thinking that these statistics do not apply to you? Think again! The term "coronary artery diseases" includes everything from high blood pressure, blood clots, blocked arteries (high cholesterol, LDL, triglycerides can cause this) to an actual stroke or heart attack. Fifty percent of heart attacks happen to patients without past history of coronary artery disease. In the year 2001, more females died of CAD than of uterus, cervical, or ovarian cancers combined.

As a woman, you are already at a higher risk for being undiagnosed or untreated for your CAD. Historically, women have often not been taken seriously when they have complained of chest pain. Often chest pain was thought to be due to stress.

Sandy came into the office complaining of some shortness of breath while hiking in Colorado. Sandy also mentioned that she had felt some increased shortness of breath during intercourse. Although she had no known risk factors and was only 52 years old, we decided to check out her heart anyway. After the stress test was positive for blockage, it was determined that the best treatment was open heart bypass surgery. Sandy recovered well and made lifestyle changes to help control her blood pressure and cholesterol in order to decrease her risk for further artery blockage.

*To calculate your personal risk for coronary artery disease, do the Framingham 10-year risk calculator at www.nhlbi.nih.gov/guidelines/cholesterol/atp3xsum.pdf.

Sandy moved out of state, but we saw her recently when she was back for a visit; she came to our office to update us on her heart disease. Evidently she had gone to establish her care with a heart doctor in her new town. The doctor asked Sandy if she was having any chest pain. "No," Sandy responded. The doctor response was, "Well, then you don't have heart disease," and said that if she had never had chest pain he was certain that she never had heart disease. Sandy responded by saying, "But I have had open heart surgery." The doctor responded, "For what?" Sandy exclaimed, "For my heart disease!" It is important to remember that chest pain* is the number one symptom that you will feel with CAD. You may also have symptoms that are not typical. These atypical symptoms include shortness of breath (with walking, exercise, or even at rest), chest heaviness, shoulder pain, or unexplained and/or persistent dizziness.

Screening tests can help to rule out cardiac disease as a cause of your symptoms. For increased risk factors, screening tests include an electrocardiograph (EKG), treadmill, or lab tests. Your lab tests should include fasting lipid levels, and a homocysteine levels (you may also want a C-reactive protein that shows inflammation, which may be a CAD risk factor), and if these are elevated, you are at increased risk for CAD.

The lipid level tests should include the "bad" lipids (cholesterol, low density lipoprotein (LDL), and triglycerides) and the "good" cholesterol (high density lipoprotein (HDL)). The higher your LDL, and the lower your HDL, the higher your risk is for CAD. As a female, a screening EKG may not be accurate and will sometimes appear falsely positive for blockage. If your EKG appears positive, you may need an echocardiograph (echo) or nuclear imaging (using an injected dye to look at blood flow in your arteries).

There is also the coronary calcium calcification tests. Normal arteries should not have calcification. If you have calcification-plaque in you arteries, you are at higher risk for a stroke or heart attack. The higher your score, the higher your risk for a CAD event. This test does not show blockage, narrowing, or artery spasm.

The "gold standard" test for assessment of coronary heart disease (when the other tests may only indicate blockage) is an angiogram. During this test you will have a tube inserted into your groin, and while dye is injected, the doctor uses a special X-ray while watching a screen for any blockage. If blockage is found, the doctor can often remove it by placing a stent to open the artery. If the heart disease is too extensive, you may need open-heart bypass surgery. What are your risk factors for coronary artery disease? Please take a minute to take the survey on this page. The life you save may be your own

*All chest pain should be evaluated

Your Personal Risk Assessment for Coronary Artery Disease

	YES	NO
• Are you 55 years old or older?	____	____
• Do you smoke?	____	____
• Have you had a first-degree relative diagnosed with CAD before 55 years of age?	____	____
• Do you mainly eat foods that are higher in sugar, salt, fat, or animal products?	____	____
• Do you avoid eating fruits and vegetables?	____	____
• Are you frequently emotionally stressed?	____	____
• Do you exercise less than 3 times a week?	____	____
• Are you 20 or more pounds overweight?	____	____
• Do you drink more then 2 alcoholic drinks a day?	____	____
• Do you take birth control pills or estrogen?	____	____

After lab testing answer these:	YES	NO
• Is your cholesterol higher than 200 mg/dl?	____	____
• Is your HDL lower than 40 mg/dl?	____	____
• Is your blood pressure higher than 130/85?	____	____
• Are your trigylcerides higher than 150 mg/dl?	____	____
• Is your LDL higher than 130 mg/dl?	____	____
• Is your fasting blood sugar higher than 110 mg/dl?	____	____

If you answered "yes" to any of the questions, then you have a wonderful opportunity to make lifestyle changes that can lessen your risks and help prevent coronary artery disease. Your new goal should be to have a healthy and powerful heart every day of your life so you can enjoy every glorious day. If you don't make changes now, then when? If you don't do it for yourself, who will? If not for yourself, do it for your partner, kids, and family. You can do it!

Be heart smart, healthy and prevent heart disease: Start today

Lipid Control:
>   Your lipid goals should be:
>>   Cholesterol less than 200 mg/dl
>>   LDL less then 130 mg/dl (less than 100 mg/dl if CAD or diabetes)
>>   Triglycerides less than 150 mg/dl
>>   HDL greater than 45 mg/dl

Blood Pressure Control:
>   Maintain BP that is less than 130/85 mg

Blood Sugar:
>   Average less than 110 mg/dl

Energize with Exercise:
>   Exercise 5 times a week for 30 minutes

Daily Nutrition:
>   (See "Enjoy Your Life" chapter)
>>   Eat 5 fruits and veggies, take a multivitamin, eat 25 grams of fiber, drink
>>   64 oz of water, limit fat/salt/sugar intake, and limit alcohol intake to less
>>   than 4 oz wine, 12 oz of beer, or 1.5 oz of liquor per day.
>>   Do not use estrogen to prevent CAD
>>   Do not smoke
>>   Consider taking 81 mg of aspirin a day if okayed by your doctor
>>   Maintain a healthy weight
>>   Consume less than 300 mg of cholesterol daily
>>   Choose chicken, turkey, lean cuts of red meat, fish (salmon, sardines, trout, tuna), low-fat
>>   dairy, olive or canola oil

Simply walking a total of three hours per week can decrease your risk of stroke or heart attack by 40 percent! It is felt that 30 percent of strokes and heart attacks are due to lack of exercise.

It doesn't matter what type of exercise—just get your body moving! Whether you walk, run, or do your favorite exercise, you get cardiac benefits. Exercise decreases blood pressure, risk for cancers and diabetes, and improves weight maintenance. So get started today!

Tips for a Healthy Lifestyle:

- Be active: move your body! Exercise 3–5 times a week, 30 minutes each time.
- Be happy: surround yourself with your "fans." Avoid people who give you side effects when you are around them.
- Eat what you enjoy: but limit yourself to one serving size.
- Eat breakfast: start your metabolism's engine to burn calories more efficiently.
- Take one multivitamin a day that has folic acid, and vitamins E, A, and C.
- Take one 81 mg coated aspirin every day (if okayed by your doctor).
- Enjoy yourself: life is a gift.
- Make healthy food choices: choose less sugar, fat, and salt. Choose more fruits, vegetables, and grains (at least 5 times a day).
- Maintain a healthy weight.

Notes: Avoid extreme dieting (increased or decreased amounts of one food category) because it can increase LDL, thereby increase CAD. Fat and sugar eaten are stored as fat. Cholesterol is made from this stored fat. Decrease fat and sugar consumption. For every one pound you lose, you lose two points in cholesterol. Folic acid helps to decrease homocysteine levels that when elevated can contribute to heart blockage.

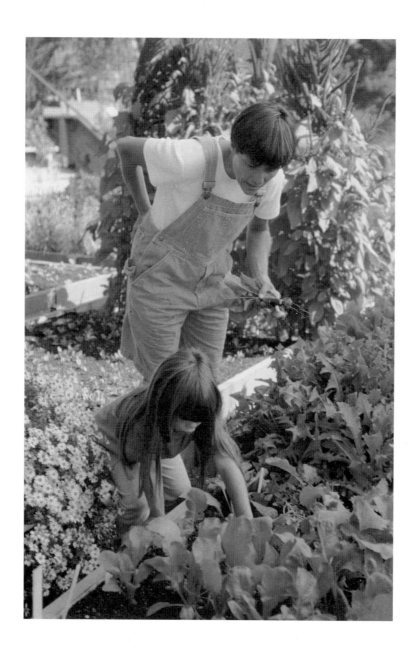

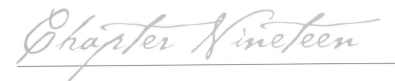

Chapter Nineteen

Forty percent of all females over 50 years old will get an osteoporosis fracture. After you have had your first fracture, you have a fivefold increase in your chances of getting a second fracture.

Chapter 19: Osteoporosis The Silent Destroyer

My next patient was new to me, and I noticed in the nurse's notes that she was here to be seen for back pain. As I entered the examination room, I noticed the patient was sitting in the visitor's straight-backed chair instead of on the examination table. I asked the patient to tell me about her back pain and when it started. She replied that it happened as she was preparing a meal and had gone to the refrigerator, opened the door, and bent over to lift an item from the shelf. She heard a loud snap and felt an instant and unbearable pain in her middle back area. Sure enough, X-rays confirmed she had fractured a vertebrae in her back simply by bending over to get something out of the refrigerator. Now she had disabling pain and had lost the freedom to do her daily tasks because of her vertebrae fracture. Imagine, with a simple bend of the waist, a disabling fracture strikes and completely changes the life of an unsuspecting victim. With a simple flexion of the waist, this woman now has to compromise what activities she chooses, and has less freedom than she previously enjoyed. Yet had she had a bone density test and/or assessment for her risk factors for fracture, this may have been prevented.

In 1995, approximately 13.8 billion dollars were spent in the United States on managing hip fractures (or 32,000 dollars per hip fracture). As you start to get older and your longevity increases, you can expect to have an increased risk for a fracture. The longer you live, the more chance you have of suffering from a hip fracture in your lifetime. **Osteoporosis is one of the most serious—and most preventable— health issues facing you.** Seventy percent of all females over 80 years of age have osteoporosis. The effects of osteoporosis on your body can be diminished if you start to be evaluated to determine your risks for hip fracture or vertebral fracture and you start preventive measures before menopause. If you have risk factors, you may need a bone density done before menopause. Otherwise, if you have no risk factors or known lifestyles that could cause osteoporosis, you could be tested at age 65. If you have increased risk factors, family history of osteoporosis, or if you have had a non-traumatic fracture after age 25, you may want to get a screening bone density test at or before menopause.

This is one of those exciting areas of medicine where you can make a tremendous difference in your future morbidity and freedom with early risk assessment and a few small adjustments to your current lifestyle. Osteoporosis is one of those areas of medicine where prevention can have a significant impact on your future.

If you do not start taking care of yourself, who will? The choice is yours to live a better and healthier life. We hear the word osteoporosis and most of us immediately think of fractures, stooped posture, and getting shorter. The stooped posture you witness in relatives and loved ones is also related to osteoarthritis and degenerative joint disease that causes us to lose the disc space between the vertebrae. The effects of osteoporosis cause our bones to wedge and deform, leading to stooped posture and height loss. In your 30s you may have been 5-foot-7 inches tall, but in your 70s you are down to 5-foot-4 inches tall—due to the effects of osteoporosis.

What exactly is osteoporosis? As you grow and develop (up to about age 34) your body continues to form bone density to keep your body's bones solid and strong. From age 34 to menopause your body relies on this bone density to keep the bone that has been previously formed in your body remaining strong. For most, the bones do stay nice and strong for years—that is, until menopause. At menopause you start to lose bone density and become susceptible to fractures and decreased vertebral height thus causing you to lose inches in your height. Forty percent of all females over 50 years old will get an osteoporosis fracture. After you have had your first fracture, you have a fivefold increase of getting a second fracture. For the first five years after menopause you lose up to 20 percent of your bone density because of the decreased estrogen production by your ovaries.

Estrogen is one way to help prevent osteoporosis, but as recent studies show, estrogen may not be the best first choice to prevent or treat osteoporosis; you can also take calcium with vitamin D, do weight bearing exercises, eat calcium-rich foods, or consider taking a bisphonate medicine that helps to prevent to prevent/treat osteoporosis. As the ovaries decrease the production of estrogen, the bones start to look moth eaten and weakened in architecture. This early, silent change to weaker bones is called osteopenia. Osteoporosis is the next stage that happens as you continue to lose bone density. Osteoporosis is where there are holes and fragile pillars in your bone structure; the bones become so fragile in severe osteoporosis cases that by simply bending over or sneezing too hard you could break a vertebrae!

With osteoporosis, the most common fracture risk sites are the hip, vertebra spine, wrist, forearm, and rib. Think of a normal bone as pound cake, think of osteopenia as sponge cake, and think of osteoporosis as an angel food cake. The pound cake can resist pressure and weight placed upon it; whereas, the angel food cake easily collapses and falls with the least amount of pressure or stress.

Are you at risk for this silent, disabling disease? Fortunately, the results from the National Osteoporosis Foundation Risk Assessment Study are now completed and will help you determine your personal risk for osteoporosis. According to this study, your risk factors for vertebral and hip fractures can be looked at on a very personal level. The wonderful thing about identifying your risk is you can probably change your future, allowing yourself the freedom from the burden of fractures.

Your risk of this silent disease statistically says that 1 out of 2 women with osteoporosis— you or a friend—will get an osteoporosis fracture in your lifetime. Twenty four percent of the time, if you get a hip fracture, you could die within one year after your hip fracture.

What if you get a vertebral (spine) fracture? You have a 1 in 5 chance that you will have another vertebral fracture within five years. If you happen to be 50 years old, white, and postmenopausal, your chance of dying from your hip fracture is similar to that of breast cancer. If you don't die of your hip fracture in the first year, 30 percent of the time if you have had a hip fracture you will end up in a long-term care facility; and if you *do* have that hip fracture, there will be a 50 percent chance that you will be disabled long term.

What are your personal risk factors for this silent disabling disease? Listed on the following page are your personal risk factors that could possibly increase or decrease your chances of getting osteopenia, osteoporosis and disabling fractures in your future.

Your Personal Risk Assessment for Osteoporosis

These increase your risk for osteoporosis:

	YES	NO
• Are you older than 65 years of age?*	____	____
• Do you have a personal history of adult fracture (non-traumatic)?*	____	____
• Do you have a maternal family history of osteoporosis or osteopenia?	____	____
• Are you Caucasian, Asian or Hispanic heritage?*	____	____
• Do you smoke?*	____	____
• Are you considered underweight?*	____	____
• Do you exercise less than three times a week?	____	____
• Do you have a history of frequent dieting?	____	____
• Do you consume less than 800 mg of Calcium a day?	____	____
• Have you used steroids more than three times a year or more than three months at a time?	____	____
• Do you drink more that 20 oz. of caffeine a day?	____	____
• Do you use thyroid hormones?	____	____
• Do you use a diuretic?	____	____
• Do you consume more than 8 oz. of alcohol in a week?*	____	____
Osteoporosis Increased Risk Total	____	____

Note: The more "yes" answers, the higher your risk is for osteoporosis.

*"Yes" answers to these items put you at an even higher risk for osteoporosis.

These will decrease your risk for osteoporosis:

	YES	NO
• Do you do weight bearing exercise greater than three times a week?	____	____
• Do you use estrogen supplementation?	____	____
• Do you consume more that 1200 mg of calcium a day if premenopausal?	____	____
• Do you consume more than 1500 mg of calcium a day if you are postmenopausal?	____	____
• Are you African-American?	____	____
Osteoporosis Decreased Risk Total	____	____

Note: The more "yes" answers, the lower your risk is for osteoporosis.

All information above adapted with permission from "AACE Osteoporosis Guidelines." *Endocrinology Practice* 7, no. 4 (2001): 1–19.

Everyday, you need to be practicing prevention by taking 1200 mg (1500 mg if postmenopausal) of calcium with vitamin D (unless your diet alone can supply this amount). Vitamin D assists in the absorption of calcium. In addition, your body does not absorb more than 500 mg of calcium at a time very well; therefore, you need to take your calcium two to three times a day.

When looking for calcium supplements, consider a source that has 500–600 mgs of calcium per pill and has vitamin D supplementation. You can also add calcium-rich foods to your diet, do weight-bearing exercise for 30 minutes, daily, walk, and do weight resistance exercises. To help maintain your current bone density, use 3–5 pound weights and do 12 repetitions of each exercise, alternating days for upper and lower body. You might be asking yourself if you should be getting a bone mineral density study in your 30s or 40s to see how strong your bones are; if you did get a screening bone density in your 30s or 40s, it would probably look normal unless you had increased risk factors. This normal value would give you a false sense of security that you aren't currently—and won't be—at a risk for osteoporosis. But remember, 20 percent of all bone mass, or density, is lost during the first five years after menopause. So you may look normal now, but this silent destroyer may affect you two years after menopause despite how great your bone density looked or how few risk factors you had in your 40s.

Most women have their last period around 51 years old. If you do not have any spotting or bleeding for six months after (what you think is) your last period, you are probably in menopause. After this point, you are then what is called postmenopausal. Menopause may be a good time to get a bone density test done if you have increased risk factors. All women 65 years old should have a bone density test if they haven't had one already.

A bone density test is considered to be the best predictor of your future risk for fracture. The "gold standard" by which to measure bone mineral density is called the dual-energy X-ray absorptionmetry or (DEXA). This machine measures your bone mineral density at your hip and vertebral spine. Your wrist, phalanx, or heel measurement can be done by a machine called peripheral-dual energy X-ray absorptionmetry or (pDEXA). The pDEXA measures the distal sights of your body and correlates fairly well with the "gold standard" DEXA. The pDEXA is the machine most commonly used for screening of bone mineral density; this is the machine you see being used at the mall, family practice clinics, and health fairs. When the pDEXA is done of an extremity does **not** predict a hip fracture as well as a DEXA of the hip does. So if you want to know your hip fracture risk, you would be better off having a DEXA to assess your bone mineral density. There is also a single X-ray called the SXA, which is an ultrasound of the heel.

Who should have a DEXA performed? Some women with risk factors who are in their first years of menopause may benefit from having a DEXA screening. In addition, any women over 65 years would benefit from a DEXA screening. Also all adult women—regardless of age, with history of non-traumatic fracture or history of steroid use longer than three months—should have a bone density screening. Also, women who are considering treatment and need confirmation of osteoporosis and women who have been on long-term HRT who need to consider other options should be screened with a bone density. If you are postmenopausal and have had a recent history of a bone fracture, you should discuss with your doctor about getting a DEXA performed to assess your further risk factors, prevention and treatment choices.

Interpreting Your Bone Density Test Results

If you decide to get a DEXA or a pDEXA how do you interpret your results? Bone mineral density scores are based on the World Health Organization criteria and compares your results to a healthy, premenopausal, white young adult female between the age of twenty and twenty-two years old. The results are given as a "T-score:"

T-score:	0	(normal) is equal to a healthy, premenopausal, young, white female.
T-score:	-1 to -2.5*	is osteopenia. This rating means you have double the risk of getting a fracture compared to a healthy, premenopausal, young, white female.
T-score:	-2.5	and greater is classified as osteoporosis. This rating means you have four times the risk of getting a fracture compared to a healthy, premenopausal, young, white female.

*If your "T-score" is -1.5 and you have risk factors, you need to consider treatment. If your "T-score" is -2.5 or greater (with or without risk factors), you need treatment.

Tips for Osteoporosis Prevention

- Take 1200 mg to 1500 mg of calcium with vitamin D daily. To absorb calcium you need vitamin D. If you are younger than 50 years old, you need 200 international units (IU) of vitamin D daily. If you are 51 to 70 years old, you need 400 IU of vitamin D daily. If you are older than 71, you need 600 IU of vitamin D daily.
- Eat foods rich in calcium, daily.
- You need to exercise 30 minutes daily; walking and weight-resistant exercises are a perfect choice.
- Evaluate your home and work environment: prevent falls by buying good shoes, having good sight and hearing, and wearing fitted, solid, low-heeled shoes. Have intact stairways, handrails, good lighting, and no throw rugs.
- Drink less than 8 ounces of caffeine per day. Caffeine is a diuretic and makes you urinate more often. The more you urinate, the more you urinate out the calcium you are taking in.

If you're not an "exerciser" and are afraid of exercising because you don't want to "bulk up"—don't think of exercise in those terms. Think of exercise as getting fit and toned. **Think of it as strength-training to avoid a fracture in the future. Exercise helps you maintain your freedom of mobility and strength. Exercise helps you remain agile, flexible, and to maintain your balance. Exercise also gives you the freedom to be "spur of moment" and to partake in any type of physical activity your heart desires such as taking a bike ride with your kids, walking up a cliff to view a beautiful sunset with a loved one, or swimming with a friend. Regular exercise allows you to have the flexibility, strength, and conditioning to live your life to the fullest.**

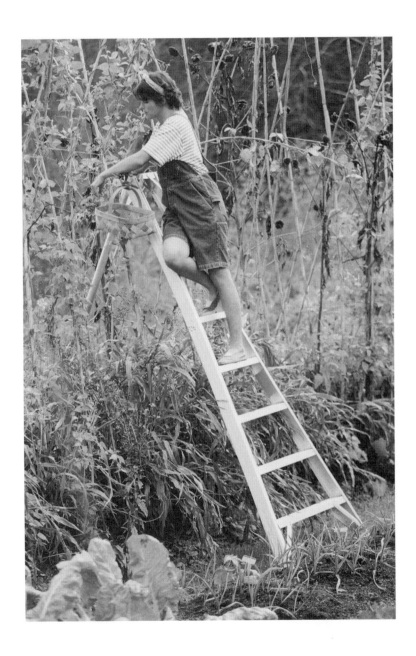

If your bone density test shows you have osteoporosis, you will have several treatment choices. These treatment choices include estrogen, alendronate (Fosamax), raloxifene (Evista), risedronate (Actonal) and calcitonin. Please see the chart below for treatment choices, known benefits, and potential side effects.

	Osteoporosis Treatment Choices		
Type	Route	Benefits	Side Effects
Estrogen*	Prevent: daily oral or patch	Increases bone mineral density in spine and hip, lowers cholesterol, LDL, and increases HDL.	Breast tenderness. Needs progesterone taken with it if uterus present. Increases gallstones, blood clots, strokes, and heart attacks. Bone loss occurs if stopped taking. Breast cancer higher if used for 4+ years. Increases triglycerides.
Fosamax (alendronate) "bisphosphonate"	Prevent: tablet 5 mg or 35 mg once weekly Treat: 10 mg daily or 70 mg once weekly	Increases bone mineral density in hip and spine. Decreases spine, hip wrist, rib, arm, and pelvis fractures.	GI upset. Esophagus or stomach ulcers. Binds to food so must take in a.m. fasting with 8 oz water and remain upright for 30 min. after taking. Calcium supplements may interfere w/ absorption so space doses.
Actonel (riserdronate) "bisphosphonate"	Prevent or treat: tablet 5 mg daily or 35 mg weekly tablet	Increases bone mineral density in hip, spine, hip, wrist, rib, arm, and pelvis fractures. May decrease spine fractures in first year of taking.	GI upset. Esophagus or stomach ulcers. Binds to food so must take in a.m. fasting with 8 oz water and remain upright for 30 min after taking. Calcium supplement may interfere with absorption so space doses.
Miacalcin (calcitonin-salmon) "hormone bone reabsorption inhibitor"	Treat: nasal spray one spray each a.m. alternate nostrils daily. Take calcium (1500 mg w/vitamin D), daily. To use must be 5 years postmenopausal.	Increases bone mineral density to spine.	Joint discomfort, nose irritation, headache
Evista (raloxifene) "selective estrogen receptor modulator" (SERM)	Prevent and treat: tablet 60 mg daily	Increases density of spine. Lowers bone reabsorption. Overall reduction in breast cancer. Lowers cholesterol and LDL.	3 times higher risk of blood clots. Hot flashes (so wait to take until menopausal hot flashes decrease). Leg cramps

*The recent Women's Health Initiative (WHI) study shows that estrogen may not be your first choice for prevention or treatment for osteoporosis.

Note: Future (not yet FDA approved) treatment choices include fluoride and parathyroid hormone (increases bone formation and lowers risk of non-spine fracture), and new surgery techniques that increase bone strength.

© 2002 Dr. Robin Hartley

Recommended Daily Calcium*

	Age	Calcium mg per day
	9–18 years	1,300
	19–50 years	1,000–1,200
	50+ years	1,200–1,500

Good Calcium Sources*

Dairy	Serving Size	Calcium Content (mg)
Milk (skim to 3% fat)	1 cup	300
Yogurt	1 cup	240–400
Ice cream	1/2 cup	100
Cottage cheese	1/2 cup	100
American cheese	1 slice	200
Swiss cheese	1 slice	270
Other Sources		
Sardines (w/ Bones)	3 oz.	370
Salmon (canned w/bones)	3 oz.	210
Broccoli	1 cup	180
Egg	1 medium	55
Soybean (tofu)	4 oz	155
Orange juice (w/calcium)	6 oz	200
Bok choy	1 cup	250
Collard greens	1/2 cup	170
Cabbage	1 cup	65
Sesame seeds	1/2 cup	580
Almonds	1/2 cup	150
Cooked spinach	1 cup	165
Squash	1 cup	55
Cooked beans	1/2 cup	90
Dried figs	1/2 cup	270
Pudding (with milk)	1/2 cup	130
Pancake	4 inches	58
Tortilla	6 inches	60

Commonly Used Calcium Supplements*

Type	Calcium (mg)	Dose (tablets)
Caltrate	600	1 twice a day
	600+vitamin D	1 twice a day
	600 plus chewables (vitamin D)	1 twice a day
Calcium carbonate (40 percent)	600	1 twice a day
Citracal	500	1 twice a day
	250 plus	4 a day
One-a-day (bone strength)	500 mg+vitamin D+soy	1 twice a day
(calcium plus)	500 mg+vitamin D+magnesium	1 twice a day
Os-Cal	500 mg+vitamin D	1 twice a day
Viactiv chewable	500 mg+vitamin D	1 twice a day

*Check bottle label to get 500–600 mg per tablet. If vitamin D is not listed, you need to add 400 mg of vitamin D supplement or a multivitamin with vitamin D. Calcium pills can be large; if you have difficulty swallowing pills, consider chewable, gelcap, or liquid forms of calcium supplements.

Note: Most of the information on this page is adapted from "AACE Osteoporosis Guidelines" Endocrinology Practice 7, no. 4 (2001): 301, 304, 305.

To view a bone from a **normal**, 75-year-old female, see photo **5d**; to view a bone from a 47-year-old female with an **osteoporotic fracture**, see photo 5c.

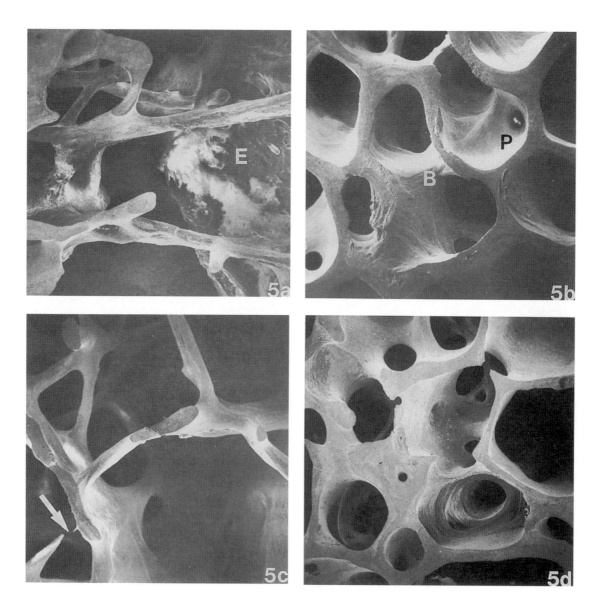

FIG. 5. Low power scanning electron micrographs of iliac crest biopsies from two osteoporotic females, aged 61 and 47 years, respectively, with multiple vertebral compression fractures (a and c), and autopsy samples from a 44-year-old normal male (b) and a 75-year-old normal female (d) who had suffered sudden death. Note that the lack of trabecular bone in the biopsy shown in (a) allows a clear view of the endosteal surface (E) of one of the cortices. P, trabecular plate; B, trabecular bar. Field width = 2.6 mm in each case.

Osteopenia and Osteoporosis Questions

Question #1: How do I know if I need calcium?
Answer: First of all, every day may have a different or correct answer depending on your diet for that day. Your daily goal should be 1200 mg (1500 mgs if postmenopausal) of calcium a day. Remember to take calcium with vitamin D, 2–3 times a day for best absorption.

Question #2: I drink lots of milk, do I really need to take additional calcium?
Answer: I find that most women who are calorie counting won't drink the six glasses of milk required a day to get to the 1200 milligrams. So, look at your daily intake of calcium and if it is below 1200 milligrams then you probably do need an additional calcium supplement with vitamin D.

Question #3: Can't I use a chewable antacid?
Answer: Probably not. First of all, you would have to chomp down part of a roll every day. Secondly, calcium is best absorbed with vitamin D, and most chewable antacids do not have vitamin D. Thirdly, calcium is best absorbed in an acidic stomach. And what do antacids do? They nullify the acid of your stomach therefore making it difficult to absorb the calcium in the antacid tablet.

Question #4: Why would osteopenia or osteoporosis even happen to me?
Answer: You lose 20 percent of your bone mass in the first five years after menopause. With menopause, estrogen levels decrease and this causes cells to take away your bone mass so you end up with thin, brittle, easily breakable bones. Statistics show that you or your best friend (if you or they have osteoporosis) will have a major osteoporotic bone fracture in your lifetime after age 50. So, a small amount of prevention now can reap huge rewards during postmenopause.

Question #5: I had a bone density test and it showed osteoporosis and I've started my treatment. When should I have a repeat DEXA?
Answer: You should have a repeat DEXA in one to two years to assess that the treatment is working and that your bone density is being maintained. Then, repeat occasionally to confirm the effectiveness of your treatment.

Question #6: Is just taking calcium and exercise enough?
Answer: Only if you have a normal bone mineral density measured by a DEXA. **This silent destroyer may still be chipping away your bones without you even knowing it until you have that unexpected fracture.** Taking calcium alone can slow the bone loss, but there is still a gradual loss of the bone. Women who seem to do the best are women who take calcium and estrogen, or calcium and a bisphosphonate.

Question #7: I had a bone density done and it showed levels that were osteopenia and osteoporosis. When is the best time to start treatment?
Answer: Maybe right away. The National Osteoporosis Foundation recommends treatment of osteoporosis. Osteopenia needs to be treated if you have increased risk factors. The worse the score for your bone mineral density and the more risk factors you have, the greater the lifelong benefit of treating osteopenia so you can continue being strong and empowered.

Question #8: What if, after taking bone medicine for two years, my DEXA shows no change or even a slight decrease in my bone mineral density?
Answer: This does not indicate treatment failure. Your treatment should continue. Just imagine: you would probably have been much worse off without any treatment at all. At least now you've almost maintained your previous bone density.

Question #9: How often should I get a DEXA?

Answer: You should consider getting a baseline at menopause if you have increased risks, or at least at age 65, even if you have no risk factors. If you have normal bone mineral density, you can check every three to five years. If you're in a prevention program, check your bone mineral density every two years until the bone mass is stable, and then every two to three years. If you're in a treatment program, check every year until bone mass is stabilized and then every two years.

Question #10: Why should I even bother to take extra calcium?

Answer: Put simply, if you fall, you do not want to get a hip fracture because you will not be able to get up with your hip fracture; and, most importantly, you want to be able to live your life fully in a spontaneous way. You want to be able to play tennis, golf, walk, run with your kids and grandkids, and **remain in charge of your body and your life and not sit disabled on the sidelines in the sunset of your years. It is a gift of freedom. You need to be active; you're going to live one-third of your life after menopause.**

Live it up, be free, dream, thrive. Make good decisions now to prevent this disease. Allow yourself to be your best and to celebrate every year with freedom, agility, strength, and power.

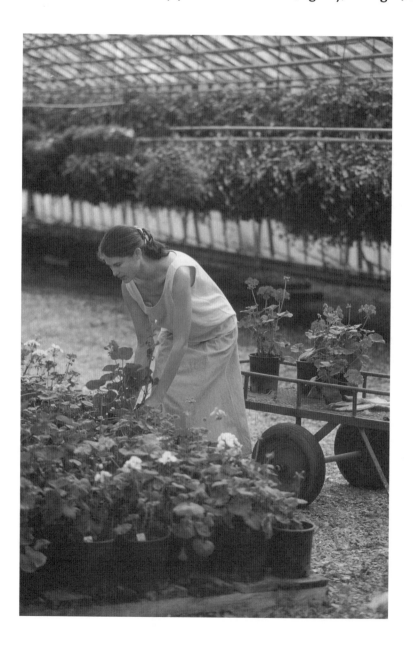

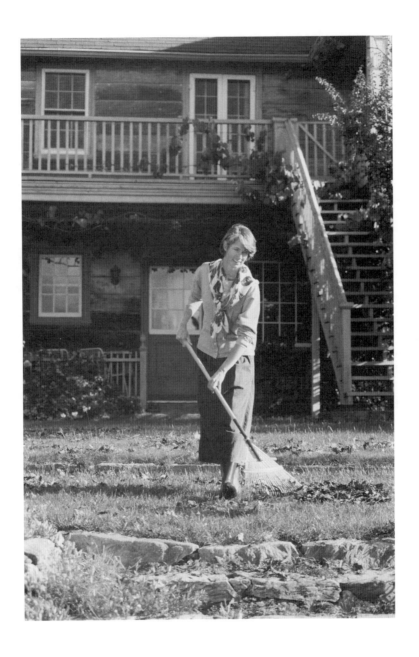

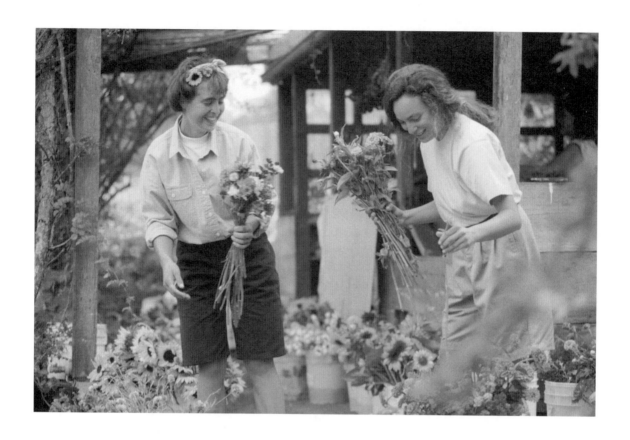

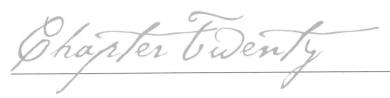

Chapter Twenty

Urinary incontinence and your selection of treatment comes down to an issue of quality of life. Do you want to be the one who always has to say "no" to social outings for fear that you will embarrass yourself with leakage in a public place?

Chapter 20: Don't Make Me Laugh, or... I'll Have to Cross My Legs

One of my 65-year-old patients, when asked about urinary incontinence or "accidents," proudly announced to me she had never used a public restroom in all of her adult years—never! Can you imagine? There should be an award for this accomplishment, or better yet, an award for the leg crossing, controlled sneezing, and body contortion she must go through to prevent any leakage when she laughs, coughs, sneezes, or waits too long.

My patient Sally, on the other hand, can tell you the quickest path to any bathroom location within a 100-mile-radius of her home. Most events she participates in would not be complete if she did not pre-plan a restroom break before departure, estimate her beverage intake during the event, and assess her seat location and its proximity to the closest restroom. Every road trip requires the mapping of streets to get to the destination and the additional "bathroom mapping."

Sally's bathroom mapping to the grocery store includes planning the fastest route to the store—and once inside the store doors—how many paces to the closest restroom. The new "super stores" or large convenience stores are a bit more of a challenge. Sally has to plan her bathroom mapping around her shopping: first to cards and cosmetics, and then back to soaps and detergents to be near the restroom just in case she needs to go to "freshen up" before the long checkout line and the car ride home.

Urinary incontinence is a big business. According to one survey of 7,000 women, 41 percent said they had at least one episode, a month, of urinary incontinence. Thank goodness for mini-pads and Depends. Eighteen billion dollars (yes, billion) were spent on adult diapers last year alone.

What exactly is urinary incontinence? The two most common types of urinary incontinence are overactive bladder (formerly called urinary incontinence) and stress incontinence. Overactive bladder is having to urinate more frequently than eight times in 24 hours. You have a sense of urgency and have to race to the restroom immediately or you could have leakage. With an overactive bladder, you may also awaken during the night and have to urinate.

On the other hand, stress incontinence is when you leak urine during coughing, laughing, sneezing, lifting, and/or exercise. Usually, there is only a small mount of leakage, and you can usually reach the restroom in time. You can also have a "mixed" condition, in which you have symptoms from both types.

If you have symptoms, you should see your doctor for a physical exam, urinalysis, and other testing to make sure your plumbing is working and that you evacuate your bladder completely with urination. Your doctor will review your medicines, lifestyle habits, look at your anatomy, and check for an infection or disease that could be causing your symptoms.

Signs and Symptoms

Overactive Bladder
Frequent urination
Urgency
Night awakening to urinate

Stress Incontinence
Leakage when you cough, laugh, sneeze, exercise, or lift an object

Your Personal Survey for Stress Urinary Incontinence*

	YES	NO
• Do you urinate more frequently than 8 times in 24 hours?	___	___
• Are you awakened more often than 2 times per night to go to the restroom?	___	___
• Do you have urgency (Got to go now!)	___	___
• Do you have urgency with leakage? Are you often wearing mini-pads or Depends, just in case?	___	___
• Do you find that you decrease your fluid intake away from home?	___	___
• Do you find that you do bathroom mapping, i.e. planning events and trips with restroom locations in mind-just in case?	___	___
• Do you decrease your amount of sexual relations due to possible leakage?	___	___
• Do you avoid going shopping, going out with friends or other social events due to possibility of leakage?	___	___

*If you answered "yes" to several of the above questions, you may need to see your doctor for treatment options.

Stress Urinary Incontinence

Usually, stress urinary incontinence can be treated by doing Kegel exercises. Kegels can be done while standing in the grocery store line, waiting in your car at the stop light, or talking on the phone. Follow the easy steps below to perfect your Kegel exercises.

Kegel exercises

- When you are urinating, stop your urine flow by squeezing your pelvic muscles.
- Relaxing these muscles should then allow urine flow to resume.
- If you are able to start and stop your urine flow with the muscles you are squeezing, you are using the correct muscles. If you are grunting, moaning, or grimacing while doing your Kegels, you probably need to practice your technique.
- After you have become proficient at this technique behind the closed bathroom door, you are set to do these exercises anywhere, anytime.
- Do ten sets of ten repetitions daily.
- Alternate the length of time you squeeze/hold and release with alternating short and long intervals.
- Avoid tightening the stomach, leg, or buttocks muscles at the same time.
- It may take up to three weeks to notice improvement, so be patient.

Overactive Bladder

An overactive bladder may require bladder reprogramming. This involves making yourself a schedule for planned bathroom breaks during your awake hours. If you typically run to the restroom every time you feel a twinge, you need to start using your Kegels instead until it is time for your scheduled restroom break. The idea is to space your bathroom breaks further apart. In other words, you should schedule restroom breaks throughout your day. These planned breaks should be approximately every three to four hours during your waking hours. Of course, this means giving up the IV bag of caffeine you use to get through your day. Caffeine is a diuretic and causes you to increase your frequency of urination. Also, caffeine dries your skin and tissues out—that means more wrinkles and dry hair for you. In addition, caffeine depletes your body's calcium store, so when you urinate you lose calcium; losing this calcium means you can end up osteopenia or osteoporosis, and broken bones.

In order to start your bladder reprogramming, you need to first do a urination diary. This means you write down, in a log, your urination pattern for the next 48 hours. Record the time of day, the estimated amount urinated, if you had a sense of urgency, if you had any leakage, and the estimated amount leakage (if any).

After you have analyzed your daily urination habits and patterns, you can then schedule bathroom breaks during times that make sense for you. You should schedule urination every three to four hours. Remember to decrease fluid in the evening and to decrease your caffeine intake. Also, ask your doctor about certain medications you may be taking that could be causing urinary incontinence for you. These would include diuretics, narcotics, antidepressants, antihistamines, tricyclic antidepressants, sedatives, hypertension medicines, and alcohol.

Your other treatment options for stress incontinence (other than Kegels) include pessaries (plastic tampons) inserted into the vaginal vault to push the bladder into a more upright natural position, collagen injections, electronic stimulators to the pelvic floor, alpha adnergic drugs like pseudoephedrine, topical or oral estrogen, or surgery.

For an overactive bladder, your treatment choices include behavior modifications with your bathroom diary, electronic stimulation to the pelvic floor, pulsating magnetic intervention, topical or oral estrogen, or neuro modulation by implanted electrodes. First line treatment medicines include tolterodine (Detrol La), oxybutynin (Ditropan XL), hyoscyamine (Urised), or propantheline. For mixed symptoms, you can take dicyclomine (Bentyl). Second-line treatments have slightly increased side effects; these treatments include imipramine (Tofranil) and flavoxate (Urispas). The most common side effects of these are dry mouth, constipation, visual changes, rapid heart beat, or drowsiness. These medicines are contraindicated if you have a history of GI obstruction, undiagnosed abdominal pain, glaucoma, or bladder obstruction.

Urinary incontinence and your selection of a treatment choice comes down to an issue of quality of life. Do you want to be the one that always has to say no to social outings for fear that you will embarrass yourself with leakage in a public place? Do you find yourself avoiding running errands, being with friends, participating in social events because of the possibility of accidents? Do you find when you do take road trips that you are always the one who has to stop every few miles? The more in control of your bladder you are, the more you can enjoy your day and not spend as much time circling and mapping for restrooms. Enough talk about Kegels, I've got to go...

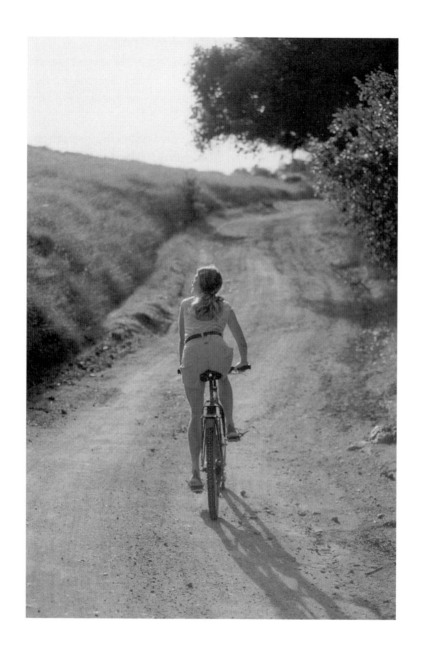

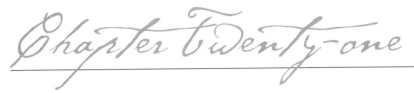

Chapter Twenty-one

If you have had a first-degree relative with a history of colon cancer, you need to do screening when you are ten years younger than they were when they were diagnosed.

Chapter 21: Colon Cancer
Scope it Out

It is probably fair to say that you have, at some point in your lifetime, noticed rectal bleeding. You probably noticed it after straining with a bowel movement and you saw bright red blood on the toilet tissue. For most of us, having constipation results from not taking time to eat our fiber cereal, fruits, and vegetables. Constipation or straining with a stool is not an uncommon scenario if you are not getting enough fiber in your diet.

At what point do you become concerned? If you notice blood with bowel movements, pain with a bowel movements, unexplained anemia, abdominal or pelvic pain, weight changes, change in your stool size—shape or color, form or frequency—you should see your doctor about scheduling a flex sigmoidoscopy (Sig)/barium enema (BE) combination or a colonoscopy to look into your colon. It used to be okay for your doctor to look with a short scope into your colon as most colon cancers were fairly close to the rectal or anal area of the colon. Now, however, colon cancer is moving up higher into the colon and is often farther away from your rectal or anal colon area, so you need a more extensive study. It has been shown that colon cancer is often related to a colon polyp that goes bad over time (usually seven years). FlexSig/barium enemas and colonoscopies allow your doctor to look in your colon for a polyp; the doctor can often remove the polyp for biopsy at the same time the scope is being performed. Therefore, your colon screening, preliminary diagnosis and polyp removal can all be done with one simple, easy, colon evacuation (called a bowel "prep" or preparation).

About the bowel prep: patients complain about the seemingly endless task of having to drink all of that bowel prep solution in order to get "cleaned out." However, if by simply drinking the bowel prep solution, taking laxatives, or taking the recommended evacuation medicine the doctor can discover and remove a precancerous polyp during a scoping procedure—then the bowel prep was worth it.

Your Personal Survey for Risk Assessment for Colon Cancer*

	YES	NO
• Do you have a first-degree relative with history of colon cancer?	___	___
• Do you have a family or personal history of ulcerative colitis, Crohn's, colitis, or familial polyps?	___	___
• Do you have a low fiber diet?	___	___
• Do you have an increased animal protein diet?	___	___
• Do you have an increased fat and refined-sugar diet?	___	___
• Are you age 50 years or older?	___	___

*The more "yes" answers, the higher your risk for colon cancer.

Your Personal Survey for Signs and Symptoms of Colon Cancer*
(Sometimes there are no symptoms)

	YES	NO
• Do you have unexplained weight loss?	___	___
• Do you have unexplained anemia?	___	___
• Do you have unexplained, recurrent rectal bleeding?	___	___
• Have you had a change in bowel movements?	___	___
• Do you have new abdominal pain?	___	___

*If you answered "yes" to any of the signs and symptoms of colon cancer, see your doctor.

Eating 25 grams of fiber and exercising for 30 minutes every day may help to decrease your risk of colon cancer. The fiber and exercise keep your bowels "moving." It is believed that the faster the stool moves through the colon, the less transit time for the stool to be in the colon; it is believed that long exposure of your colon lining to stool waste matter can change the lining of your colon causing polyps to form. These polyps can then become abnormal and change to cancer over a period of years. There is some thought that taking estrogen, aspirin, and calcium may help decrease your risk of colon cancer, but this is still being studied.

I remember one patient who came in, accompanied by a friend, after she had noticed bright red blood on the tissue paper and pain with having a stool. She was extremely anxious. I explained to her that this possibly could indicate hemorrhoids or a tear in the anal opening and that I would like to proceed by examining the area with what is called an anoscope; I explained that this is a clear, small, plastic tube, smaller than most bowel movements, that would be inserted into her anal area. The patient then became exceptionally nervous and repeatedly said she hated the idea of having this area of her body examined, and it was upsetting to her. After the patient carried on about her hating to have her anal/rectal area looked at for what seemed like an eternity, I mumbled, "Well, this doesn't make my day either." The patient paused with her complaining, and she and her friend both roared with laughter. She said she had never thought of "that end" of it (no pun intended). This completely relieved her tension, and we were able to proceed.

When should you start getting screened? Everyone should receive a screening colon test when they are 50 years of age. It is believed by some that fecal occult blood testing (FOBT) by digital rectal exam in your doctor's office, guaiac cards/hemoccult cards (those cards you take home with you to do your own stool testing on a card to be returned to the doctor), Flex Sig/barium enema, and colonoscopies are equivalent to one another. A Flex Sigmoidoscopy/barium enema is where a doctor looks at least 60 cm into your lower colon with a flexible scope and then you go to a radiology department for a barium enema and X-rays of the upper part of your colon.

A colonoscopy is where a doctor sedates you and a scope is inserted so they can look at your entire colon. Oftentimes, you can watch on a television screen as the doctor journeys through your colon with the scope. Although the guaiac/hemoccult cards and digital rectal exam by your doctor are an okay screen, they don't necessarily allow for upper colon inspection. The advantage of colonoscopy or Flex Sig is an opportunity for the doctor to visually look at the colon lining while they are examining for polyps. It also allows the doctor the option to do a biopsy or polypectomy (removing the polyp), or to give a recommendation for further evaluation.

If, however, you have increased risk factors because of personal or family history, it should be recommended that you have a colonoscopy; this is the most complete exam currently available. Current research and testing of better preps (just one pill taken to clean you out), and noninvasive CAT scan studies are currently being evaluated. Again, you should receive a screening colon test when you are 50 years of age. It is your choice whether to do a Flex Sig/barium enema or colonoscopy.

If you have had a first-degree relative with history of colon cancer, you need to do screening when you are ten years younger than they were when they were diagnosed. Anyone with unexplained rectal bleeding, rectal pain, abdominal pain, or pelvic pain may need evaluation with a colon scope. Digital rectal exam with fecal occult blood testing (FOBT) and sigmoidoscopy can be your screening tests at age 50 (start screening at age 40 if you have increased risk factors). FOBT should be done yearly, and sigmoidoscopy should be performed every three to five years. If either of the tests are positive for blood or polyps, you may need further testing. Colon cancer is the second most common cancer in the United States. Routine screening and removal of polyps can decrease colon cancer death by 80 percent.

Although colon studies are an unpleasant topic for you, and may bring a grimace to your face to even think about the exam (not to mention the prep), your colon health is important and you shouldn't ignore it. By ignoring your colon or your colon-related symptoms, or hoping your doctor doesn't have time to talk to you about it, won't make "that end" (pun intended) of your health just go away. This is one area of your health that—if you are proactive and preventive—you may be able to change for your future health and well-being. The life you save may be your own by early colon scoping and polyp removal.

Tips for Colon Health:

- You need a screening colon test starting at age 50 (age 40 if risk high factors). Screen can be fecal occult blood test and sigmoidoscopy, or colonoscopy.
- Eat a diet high in fiber, low in saturated fats, low in alcohol, and stop smoking.
- Exercise 30 minutes daily (walking is great).
- Maintain a healthy weight.
- Consider daily multivitamins with folic acid 400 mg, aspirin (if okayed by your doctor), calcium supplement (1200 mg if appropriate).
- After initial screening that is negative:
    (FOBT yearly
    Flex sigmoidoscopy and barium enema every 3–5 years
    Or colonoscopy every 5–10 years)

Questions and Answers

Question #1: I have hemorrhoids, how do I know when to be concerned?

Answer: There are countless stories of patients with hemorrhoids that didn't see their doctor because they firmly believed that their hemorrhoids were just "acting up" again. When they finally did go in to see their doctor, they found out it wasn't their hemorrhoids acting up after all—instead, they were diagnosed with colon cancer. It is always important to be checked by your doctor more frequently if you have hemorrhoids. Also, you need to report to your doctor any change in your stools such as unusual change in color, shape, or size. Also, report any changes in or worsening of your hemorrhoid symptoms. Basically, see your doctor for anything that seems unusual having to do with your bowel habits.

Question #2: Do doctors normally check in the anal-rectal area when they do a pap exam?

Answer: How can you tell what the doctor is doing "down there" with your legs in a spread eagle position, your feet locked in the stirrups, and your knees wrapped around your ears? Whether a digital rectal exam and guaiac/hemmocult cards are done during your pap or annual exam depends on your age, symptoms, and your doctor's preference of exam. Some doctors will always check the inside of the anal-rectal area to feel the back side of the uterus. Others will do a digital anal-rectal exam just to feel for polyps.

On the other hand, some doctors may not check in this area at all and will send a guaiac/hemoccult card home to look for trace blood in your stool. You collect your own stool specimen onto the card at home, and it is to be brought back to the lab to be evaluated for blood.

It is always a special treat when a patient brings their stool specimen back to our clinic in a brown paper bag and leaves the bag at the front desk saying "this is for the doctor." Then the staff, thinking that the patient has baked something special for me, leaves the bag on my desk. What an unexpected surprise I find when I eagerly open the bag to see what special goody "Mrs. Jones" has prepared for me.

Other doctors will not even address this area of your health until you are 50 years of age. At age 50, and beyond, the anal-rectal check should be a normal part of your physical and/or pap exam. Your doctor's style preference (and insurance regulations) may direct what is done during your exam. It is best to just be up front with your doctor and tell them you would like a digital rectal exam (yes, you do!), and stool card to look for hidden blood in your stool. If you have increased risk factors, suspicious symptoms, or are 50 years of age, you need to talk to your doctor about scheduling a scope study.

Question #3: Okay, you have had a scope study. When should the next testing be done?

Answer: If the scope was normal and you have no risk factors, then every five to ten years. If the scope was normal and you have risk factors, every three to five years (or sooner if warranted). If the scope was abnormal or you had polyps present (risk factors or no risk factors), you may need more frequent scope exams. Repeat the scope until it is normal and then repeat the scope every one to three years. If the scope was abnormal plus a cancer-positive polyp biopsy, you need treatment for the colon cancer and then repeat scopes as directed by your doctor. Usually every six months for three to five years and then, when normal, as determined by your doctor.

Question #4: What stool changes should I be looking for?

Answer: Some of the changes to watch for are changes in consistency, color, size, shape, and stool frequency. Change in consistency includes stools that normally were solidly formed and are now runny or very hard. Change in frequency includes if you were constipated normally, and now you are having frequent bowel movements (or you were having a bowel movement daily and you have them infrequently). Any chronic change in color, such as dark brown, black, red, or light colored should be investigated. You should investigate changes in stool size (i.e. your usual "Lincoln Logs" have now become tiny "Peanut M&M's" or runny diarrhea-type stools). The presence of blood—anything red, anytime, anywhere—should be discussed with your doctor immediately.

Question #5: What are the best sources of fiber?

Answer: Fruits, vegetables, and grains. Select a high-fiber cereal every morning to ensure you get at least a 10 mg fiber head-start for the day. Good cereal sources include All Bran and Fiber One. Actual food (versus tablets or drink) is always better because it can also provide bulk and roughage.

The best sources of fiber are vegetables, fruit, and grains. Avoid taking laxatives or stimulants. Your goal should be to eat 25 grams of fiber a day. The following are good choices:

Fruits			Veggies		
Food	**Amount**	**Fiber**	**Food**	**Amount**	**Fiber**
Apple	1 medium	3.0	Beans, baked	1/2 cup	6.0
Apricot, dried	10	2.7	Beans, green	1/2 cup	2.8
Blueberries	1 cup	3.3	Brussel sprouts	1/4 cup	3.4
Currants	1/2 cup	3.0	Carrots	1 medium	2.3
Dates, dried	10	4.2	Chick peas	1 cup	5.7
Figs, dried	10	17.0	Corn, boiled	1/2 cup	3.0
Kiwis	1 medium	2.6	Black-eyed peas	1/2 cup	3.7
Oranges	1 medium	2.9	Northern beans	1 cup	6.0
Papayas	1 medium	2.9	Kidney beans	1 cup	6.4
Peaches, dried	10 halves	10.0	Lentils	1 cup	7.9
Pears	1 medium	4.3	Lima beans	1/2 cup	7.0
Prunes, dried	10	6.0	Mixed/frozen veg.	1/2 cup	3.5
Raisins	2/3 cup	5.3	Peas	1/2 cup	3.5
Raspberries	1 cup	5.8	Potato, baked	1 medium	2.0
Strawberries	1 cup	3.9	Pumpkin	1/2 cup	3.8
			Soybeans	1/2 cup	7.5
Other			Spinach	1/2 cup	3.0
Peanuts, roasted	1/2 cup	6.0	Squash, baked	1/2 cup	2.9
Sweet potatoes	1 medium	3.4	Tomato sauce	1/2 cup	2.5

Cereals					
	Amount				
All-Bran	1/2 cup	10.0		**Breads**	
Bran Flakes	2/3 cup	5.0		**Amount**	
FiberOne	1/2 cup	13.0	Multigrain	1 slice	1.7
Raisin Bran	3/4 cup	5.0	Oatmeal	1 slice	1.9
Oatmeal, instant	3/4 cup	2.8	Wheat	1 slice	2.0
			Whole wheat	1 slice	1.6
Bran Buds	1/2 cup	8.0			
Bran Chex	2/3 cup	6.0			
Wheat bran	1/3 cup	11.0			

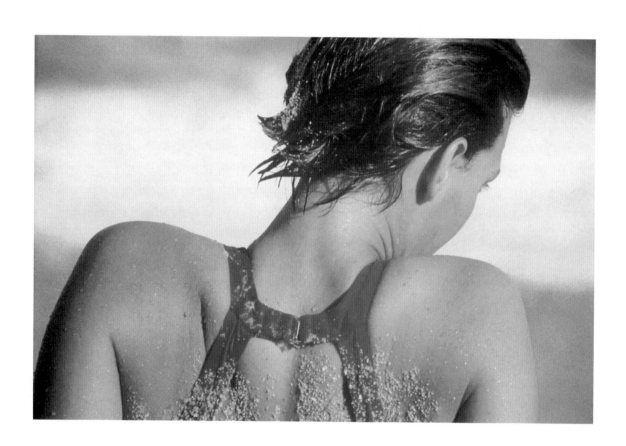

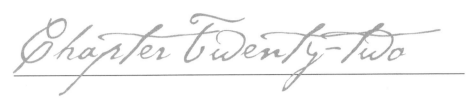

Chapter Twenty-Two

First of all, remember that SPF just buys you a little time. SPF stands for "sun protection factor." SPF 45 is not more powerful or thicker than a lower SPF. A higher SPF number just means that you are able to stay out in the sun for a longer period of time before getting a sunburn or increasing damage to your skin.

Chapter 22: The Sun Skin Cancer

Over the last few years, people have developed an idea that they look better and appear healthier if they have a tan. People tell me that they just feel better with a little added color in their skin. But remember, skin cancer can kill you. The occurrences of skin cancer will increase in epidemic proportions during your lifetime. You, yourself, have a 1 in 78 chance of getting malignant melanoma in your lifetime.

What were we thinking when we were growing up and took up sunbathing as if it were a paying summer job—lying for hours smothered in baby oil on our metallic mats? We would even adjust our mats every so often to absorb the sun's rays more efficiently. Now, because of your busy career, you enjoy the convenience of tanning beds that allow you the luxury of a quick tan—without all those wasted hours in the sun. The problem is, the ultraviolet A (UVA) rays from the tanning bed are even more harmful to your skin than the rays from the sun.

STOP NOW! With all the "sunless" tanning products on the market, there should never be a reason for you to tan again. Check out the sunless tanning products at your local department store cosmetics counter or drug store, and find the right product for you. Other than possible local skin irritation, there have been no known side effects from these sunless tanning products. Also, cosmetics companies are making bronzing powders that add radiance to your skin.

Why should you stop sunbathing or using a tanning bed? Skin cancer is caused by a lifetime of exposure to the sun. The sun has both ultraviolet B (UVB) burning rays and UVA tanning rays (tanning beds use UVA rays). The way your skin tries to protect itself against UV damage is through a tan. Tanning beds take away the initial warning (UVB or burning) that you are damaging your skin (you tan before a sunburn). Tanning beds markedly increase your risk of skin cancer. Both the sun and tanning bed cause skin cancer, wrinkles, and aging to your skin. What seems to be harmless sun exposure or an occasional sunburn sets you up for future skin cancer. **We now know that sun damage is accumulated over your lifetime and the harmful rays you received when you were 16-years-old that caused a sunburn, may (even decades later) cause skin cancer. Besides deadly malignant melanoma, you may also be at risk for squamous and basal cell types of skin cancers that can spread and possibly kill you.**

What are your risk factors for skin cancer? Remember that it is the accumulative exposure that you have received that is harmful, so answer "yes" if any apply of the items below apply to you in your lifetime.

Your Personal Risk Assessment for Skin Cancer*

	YES	NO
• Do you have a history of using a tanning bed or sun lamp?	____	____
• Do you so outdoor sports, hobbies, activities, or work?	____	____
• Do you have a family history of skin cancers?	____	____
• Are you not using sunscreen?	____	____
• Do you have light skin, or red or blonde hair?	____	____
• Have you had one severe, blistering sunburn in your youth?	____	____
• Do you have a mole that is irregularly shaped, or multicolored?	____	____
• Do you have a mole that is changing in size, shape, or color?	____	____

*The more "yes" answers, the higher your risk for skin cancer.

What are you looking for when you are trying to do a body check of your moles?

- Any mole or freckle (colored spot on the skin) that is continually scabby, irritated, or will not heal should be biopsied.
- Any mole or freckle that has changed its borders and has now become irregularly shaped, or has raised or widened in its circumference or height.
- Any mole that has changed colors or has become multicolored, or seems to be growing or enlarging.
- Any mole or freckle that looks unusual and does not appear to be like the other moles and freckles on your body.
- Any mole or freckle with any of these changes should be investigated and/or biopsied by your physician. If you are very concerned about a particular mole or freckle, ask your physician to do a biopsy or to send you to a specialist who could biopsy these areas for you. You should do full body checks every six months with a mirror. For scalp area, try using a blow dryer to expose scalp area and have a friend or partner look for abnormal patches, spots, or moles.

There are 4 warning signs for melanoma
(They are called the **ABCD**s for melanoma)

A is for **Asymmetry**:	The two halves of the mole would not match if the mole was folded in half. Instead of being round and symmetrical, each half is not a mirror reflection of itself.
B is for **Border**:	The border of the mole is irregular, scalloped, or notched instead of smooth.
C is for **Color:**	The mole color is several colors, instead of a uniform color. These colors may be black, brown, red, white, or blue.
D is for **Diameter**:	The mole diameter (width across) is larger than a pencil eraser.

Cancer Photos

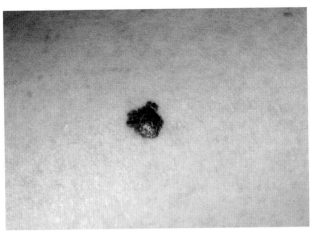

Malignant Melanoma
Irregular edge (border). Very dark.

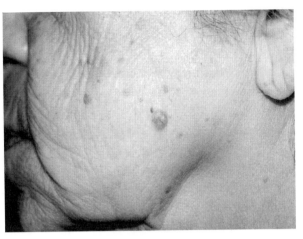

Basal Cell
Raised. Pearly color. Rolled edges.
May see tiny blood vessels in the lesion.

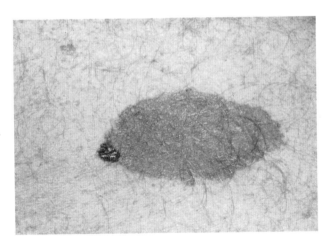

Malignant Melanoma
Irregular shape. Multicolored.

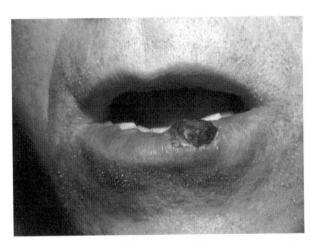

Squamous Cell
Scabby. Irritated. Slow to heal.

*Photos courtesy of Dr. Charles Love, Dermatologist, Des Moines, Iowa

Questions and Answers

Question #1: I have lots of moles and freckles. How do I even start to do checks of these moles?
Answer: You should examine yourself every six months starting from your head and continuing to your toes. Use a blow dryer to raise up your scalp hair so that a friend or your partner can look at the scalp area for abnormal moles. Any mole or freckle should be evaluated by your physician if it is suspicious looking (abnormal) or does not appear to be like the other moles or freckles on your body. If you *do* see a mole or freckle that is changed or changing, you should go to your physician as soon as possible and not wait to see if it stops changing. Time is of the essence when diagnosing and treating abnormal moles.

Question #2: What is the best sunscreen to use?
Answer: Remember, the SPF (sun protection factor) of a lotion just means that it allows you more time in the sun. SPF 45 is not more powerful or thicker than a lotion with a lower SPF. A higher numbered SPF means that you are able to stay out in the sun for a longer period of time before getting a sunburn or increasing damage to your skin. Dermatologists would say to use an SPF 45 lotion (with both UVA and UVB protection), applying 30 minutes prior to going out in the sun to allow maximum absorption into your skin, and reapplying every 30 minutes (or after swimming or a sweating-inducing activity). Remember to check the expiration date on the bottle. Buying a new bottle of sunscreen every summer means that the sunscreen will be more effective. Avoid the sun from 10:00 a.m. to 3:00 p.m. as this is the time when there is the most damaging ultraviolet (UV) light radiation. If you have to be outside, try to wear long sleeves, long pants, hats, scarves, and a SPF sunscreen and SPF lip balm to protect you from the sun.

Question #3: How long should I watch a mole or freckle that is changing?
Answer: It is best to get a skin biopsy by a trained physician when any change occurs no matter how benign the mole or freckle may appear to you. Let a pathologist look at the biopsied mole or freckle with a microscope to confirm that it is noncancerous. Ask the doctor if the margins removed from around the edges of your mole biopsy were "clean." In other words, if all abnormal cells around the area have been removed completely and the area is free of any abnormal mole or freckle cells after the biopsy.

Question #4: I have always avoided the sun, have no risk factors, and no family history of skin cancer. Is it still possible for me to get skin cancer?
Answer: To our great surprise, skin cancer is still found on people who have not been in the sun for years and have always protected their skin. In these cases, the cancer is probably related to some sunburn that they don't remember from when they were playing outdoors as a kid. It is always good to get your skin checked by your physician every six months to one year, regardless of the sun exposure that you have had in your life. Remember, even if your skin has darker pigmentation, you can still get skin cancer.

Question #5: Who is at increased risk for getting skin cancer?
Answer: Anyone and everyone is at increased risk of developing skin cancer if they have spent any time in the sun, tanning bed, or under sun lamps. Those people at highest risk are people who are blonde, redheaded, have fair skin, already have increased freckles, have a family history of skin cancer, or have a history of bad sunburn or cumulative sun exposure with lack of skin protection (clothing or lotion). Every year at your annual physical, you should ask your doctor to examine your skin for suspicious moles and freckles. Make sure that your doctor takes time to examine the back of your ears, back of your neck, and your back area. Special attention should be given to the areas you have a hard time seeing for yourself like your scalp, shoulders, back, and the backs of your legs. Also, don't forget to examine between your fingers and toes; if skin cancers are found in these areas, they can be very harmful to you.

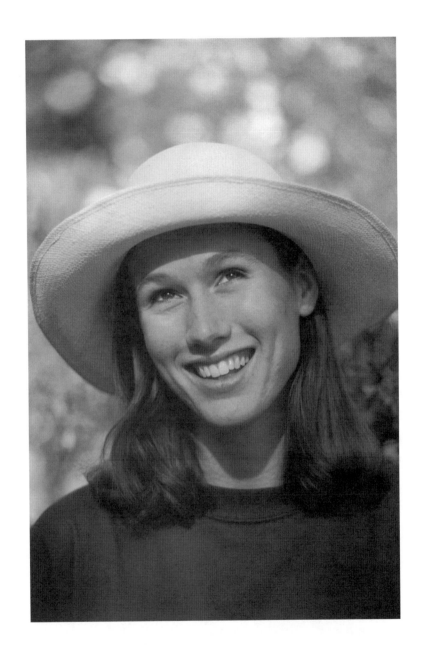

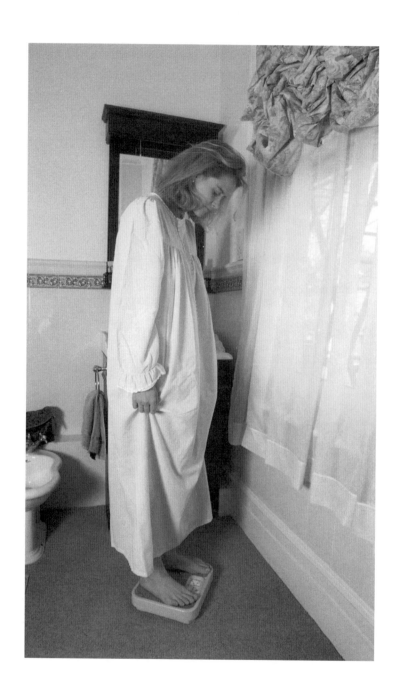

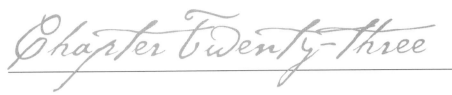

Chapter Twenty-three

Your thyroid is the body's control station for everything from sense of well-being, energy, metabolism, weight control, bowel movement, heart rate, body temperature, muscle strength, period cycles, sex drive, and skin and hair texture and moisture.

Chapter 23: Your Thyroid The Body's Control Center

A few months before Dr. Lynn Allen's first year of medical residency, she discovered she was pregnant with her second child. She had some discussion with her husband—they already had a two year old at home—about whether or not she should take that first rigorous and sleepless year of medical residency off because of her pregnancy. It was quickly decided they would be better off to get that awful first year behind them and trust that all would go well with the pregnancy.

The first year of residency was as demanding, rigorous, and exhausting as promised. In this first year, it was expected that you would sleep in the hospital every few nights so you would be available for all hospital medical questions, emergencies, and unexpected deliveries—all while working under the watchful eyes of the senior resident. These overnights were scheduled so you could be available during the night—for everything from being beeped at 2:00 a.m. about Tylenol orders for an inpatient to being startled to full alertness by a Code Blue. It was not uncommon to spend the night helping ER patients or delivering a baby. These overnights would be, of course, preceded and followed by full medical work days, going to lectures, seeing patients at the hospital and clinic, and shadowing a specialist. No wonder Dr. Allen felt tired.

It seemed her body signals were getting mixed up. Was she hungry or tired? The solution seemed to be to eat something to get more energy. Sleep became a luxury. One time she was on for a day, night, and a day—and was finally able to get off this shift to go home to meet her husband, son, and parents for a Saturday lunch. Then, the dreaded pager went off just as the ordered food was arriving to the table. A few nibbles, and Dr. Allen raced back to the hospital to assist with—what turned out to be—a surgery that lasted from mid-afternoon until midnight that night. Being seven months pregnant and having to stand in one place, helping the surgeon for seven straight hours (without so much as a bathroom or food break) is no small task. Dr. Allen made it through that shift and was finally able to rejoin her family at home early the next morning only to return back to the hospital to begin early morning rounds at 6:00 a.m.

As the first year of residency (and pregnancy) continued to march slowly on with time, she began to notice changes in her body. Dr. Allen's appetite would be vigorous. Often, one large tray of food would seem like an appetizer and a second tray of food would have to be eaten. The dry skin and thickening scalp hair must be due to the pregnancy, she figured. The big mood swings and fatigue would get better if only she could get off call for awhile and get some rest; these changes must be due to pregnancy—or all of those grueling overnight hours in the hospital, she reasoned. If only this year was over, or the baby was born, then things would be better. Dr. Allen's mother noticed these changes and asked her if they could possibly be connected with pregnancy—or perhaps a thyroid disorder? "Of course not, Mother," Dr. Allen responded. "If it was, that certainly would have been taught to us in medical school."

But her mother's words continued to echo in her mind. Could there be a connection between pregnancy and thyroid? Dr. Allen started asking her professors, mentors, and even the hospital's director of pathology if there was a connection between pregnancy and thyroid disorders. They all responded thoughtfully and shook their heads slowly responding, "No, no connection is known."

The pregnancy continued, and Dr. Allen gave birth to a beautiful baby boy. Unfortunately, the symptoms, previously attributed to pregnancy, now continued beyond the delivery. The symptoms of dry skin, coarse hair with hair loss, difficulty sleeping, moodiness, feeling like she was wearing a turtleneck sweater (when she wasn't) must all be related to the rigorous calls and overnight schedule of residency coupled with getting up through the night with a new baby or a restless two-year-old. Or, maybe Dr. Allen's first year of residency was just getting the better of her.

Finally, one day while Dr. Allen was sitting at a table and doing research in the hospital medical library, the hospital pathology director walked up and handed her a research article on a new study on what was being called "postpartum thyroiditis." It described all of the symptoms she had been experiencing. She wasn't losing her mind after all—and the residency was not getting the best of her. There was a medical reason for all the seemingly unrelated symptoms she was experiencing.

Fortunately, postpartum thyroiditis, like postpartum depression, is short-lived for most women. Postpartum thyroiditis usually lasts less than six months after the baby is delivered and doesn't usually require any medicine. There is some thought that if you have postpartum thyroiditis that you may be more prone to future thyroid abnormalities. Therefore, if you have had postpartum thyroiditis, you will want to get a TSH (thyroid stimulating hormone) drawn yearly by your doctor to monitor your thyroid.

Postpartum thyroiditis is only one type of thyroid disorder. The two most common types are hypothyroidism and hyperthyroidism. Your thyroid is the body's control station for everything from sense of well-being, energy, metabolism, weight control, bowel movement, heart rate, body temperature, muscle strength, period cycles, sex drive, to skin and hair texture and moisture.

If your thyroid is not working properly, everything seems out of sync, and you may not be able to perform at your best during daily activities. If your thyroid is sluggish and not performing well—thus not letting you perform at your best—this is called hypothyroid. **The most common symptoms of an underactive thyroid (hypothyroid) are dry coarse hair, loss of eyebrow hair, puffy face, enlarged thyroid, slow heart beat, arthritis-type symptoms, feeling cold, depression, dry skin, fatigue, forgetfulness, heavy periods, infertility, muscle aches, weight gain, constipation, and brittle nails. The causes of hypothyroidism can vary from a low iodine level in your diet, to being triggered by such things as an infection, your genetic expression, or an auto immune dysfunction.**

Hyperthyroid is an overactive thyroid and can have similar symptoms to hypothyroidism such as fatigue, depression, and moodiness. However, hyperthyroidism can have completely opposite symptoms such as thinning hair and hair loss, bulging eyes, sweating, enlarged thyroid, rapid heart beat, difficulty sleeping, heat intolerance, infertility, irritability, muscle weakness, nervousness, little to no menstrual periods, weight loss, frequent bowel movements, warm or moist palms, hand tremor, and soft nails. **After reading the symptoms of hypo- or hyperthyroid, you have to be careful not to over diagnose yourself. It can be normal for you to feel one or most of these symptoms on any given day and yet not have a thyroid disorder.**

If the symptoms of hypothyroidism or hyperthyroidism listed above describe several of the symptoms you have been feeling and these symptoms have continued to last longer than two months, you need to get a thyroid stimulating hormone level (TSH) drawn by your doctor. Most woman should get a screening TSH at age 50. If you have symptoms to suggest hypo- or hyperthyroidism, or multiple family members have a history of thyroid disorders, you may want to get a screening TSH in your 30s or 40s. Your continued lack of energy and tired feeling may be caused by a medical condition such as your thyroid.

Treatment for hypothyroidism is relatively simple and usually involves taking a daily pill of a thyroid hormone. A TSH level should be drawn yearly to make sure your dose of medicine is correct for you. Hyperthyroidism is usually treated with radioactive iodine which destroys all or part of your thyroid. Other options include taking an antithyroid pill or surgery to remove the thyroid. If you opt for the radioactive iodine treatment, this usually then makes your thyroid inactive—you become hypothyroid—and you are then given a pill of a thyroid hormone. You are then monitored by yearly blood levels of TSH and your dose is adjusted accordingly.

Once your thyroid has been treated, you should start to feel better. Hopefully, you will feel revitalized and restored enough to soar through your day full of renewed energy.

Hypothyroid
Symptoms:

Tired, fatigued
feeling cold
change in menses flow & cycle
weight gain
feeling blue, moodiness
muscles aches
constipation
dry, coarse skin, hair, nails
hoarse voice
forgetfulness

Diagnosis by:
TSH serum level
Ultrasound
If a nodule (abnormal lump)
a biopsy may be needed

Treatment:
Daily pill of thyroid hormone
Monitor TSH yearly

Hyperthyroid
Symptoms:

Tired
nervous, irritable
weight loss
rapid heart beat
easy sweating, feeling hot
frequent bowel movements
depression
muscle weakness
irregular menses
hair loss

Diagnosis by:
TSH , FT4 , ultrasound
Iodine thyroid uptake scan
If a nodule (abnormal lump)
a biopsy may be needed

Treatment:
Radioactive iodine
Surgery
Beta Blocker pill
or antithyroid pill

Thyroiditis
Symptoms:
Mixed symptoms of hypo- or hyperthyroidism

Diagnosis:
TSH, ultrasound, if needed iodine thyroid uptake scan

Treatment:
Conservative. Recheck TSH every 8-12 weeks to follow for TSH level to return to normal. TSH should be checked yearly. Thyroiditis can lead to eventual hypo- or hyperthyroidism.

Questions and Answers

Question #1: I have only a few of the symptoms listed for a thyroid disorder and these symptoms seem to come and go. Do I still need to get tested?

Answer: If these symptoms seem to be present daily (more frequently than not), and if they continue for longer than two months, it would be worth your time to see your doctor for your symptoms and to at least get a CBC (complete blood count) and a TSH.

Question #2: What if hyper- or hypothyroidism are diagnosed? Why even treat it? I certainly don't want to take a pill the rest of my life.

Answer: Over the long term, thyroid disease—if not treated—can set you up for other health issues. For example, untreated hyperthyroidism can lead to osteoporosis because of the depletion of the calcium caused by your overactive thyroid. Untreated hyperthyroidism can also cause heart arrhythmia that sets you up for an increased risk of stroke, heart attack, or a blood clot. So, if you are diagnosed with hyperthyroidism or hypothyroidism, you will want it treated so you can be your best and live a full, productive life.

Question #3: Reading over the symptoms of hypothyroidism seem to describe me—in some way—every day of my life. Should I run out to the doctor every time I feel these? How frequently should the TSH test be taken?

Answer: If you are trying to eat food that has a proper nutrition level, you are getting plenty of rest, and you are getting a good amount of daily exercise and you still feel these symptoms, you need to get a screening TSH. If that is normal, you can probably wait and be rescreened yearly or as needed. There may be a slight possibility that when you see your doctor you are in a "window of time" where your body is feeling hyper- or hypo- symptoms, but your blood level appears normal. If you are still feeling symptoms and your TSH was normal, it is best to plan a follow up visit to recheck with your doctor sooner than your next yearly physical. If your symptoms continue, you can get a TSH retested in a few months or get another type of test such as thyroid antibodies levels. Increased thyroid antibodies can show that your thyroid is affecting your own body's immune systems and you may end up being hypothyroid or hyperthyroid, or the antibodies levels may return to normal. Repeat TSH testing every six months may be warranted and treatment given if needed.

Question #4: What if you don't feel any symptoms of thyroid? Could you still have hypo- or hyperthyroidism?

Answer: Oftentimes, people with hypothyroidism (tired, dry skin, hair loss) may think that the body changes they are experiencing are completely normal during certain times of the year (such as winter); whereas with hyperthyroidism, patients can feel symptoms and discount their symptoms thinking they are just anxious, stressed, nervous, or having menopause symptoms such as hot flashes and heart palpitations.

Your doctor should check your thyroid with your yearly exam when you are 50. You may need to ask for a TSH level to be drawn after age 50 (if you are noticing thyroid symptoms as a TSH level is not routinely drawn). If you are experiencing unexplained, continued symptoms for longer than two months and you are in your 30s and 40s, you may need to ask your doctor for a TSH test.

Question #5: What if you or your doctor find a nodule or a lump in your thyroid?

Answer: If you or your doctor feels a lump or nodule in your thyroid, you may need to have a thyroid ultrasound done. If, on the ultrasound, the nodule or lump is not clearly seen as a cyst or is not consistent with hypothyroidism, then you may need further evaluation of the nodule, cyst, or lump. A thyroid cyst, nodule, or lump may need to be biopsied to confirm it is benign.

Question #6: What are the treatments for hypothyroidism or hyperthyroidism?

Answer: If you suspect hypothyroidism, your diagnosis would be confirmed by your symptoms, a TSH level, and sometimes an ultrasound. Treatment is a daily thyroid hormone replacement pill. At least yearly, TSH levels are drawn in order to adjust your pill dose, if needed.

If you suspect hyperthyroidism you would be diagnosed by your symptoms, a TSH level, Free T4, and possibly a radioactive thyroid uptake-scan to confirm an overactive thyroid. Treatment is usually with an antithyroid pill or radiation. With radiation treatment, your thyroid may become inactive-hypothyroid and you will require a daily thyroid pill. Surgery is another option, but is not as common.

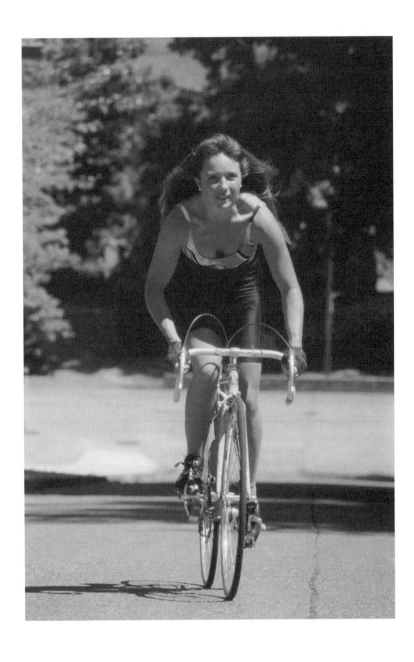

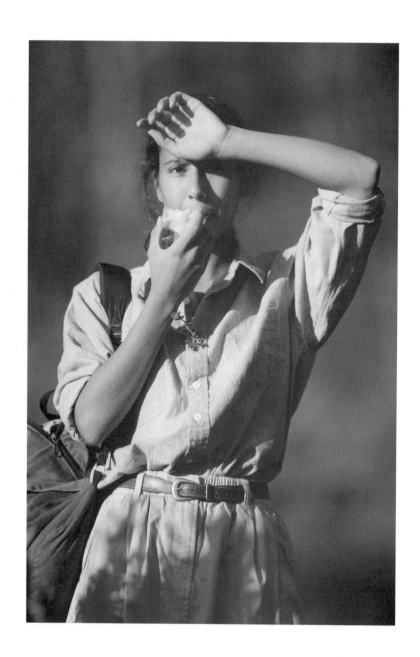

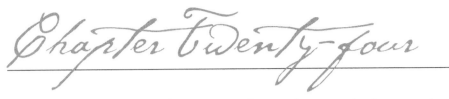

Chapter Twenty-four

With low blood sugar (or hypoglycemia), the simple acts of lying down or eating something can relieve symptoms because blood sugar flow is then restored to your brain. Your brain's fuel is blood sugar (glucose).

Chapter 24: Things that Make You Feel Shaky Blood Sugar

Dr. Lauren Warner had not lost the remaining ten extra pounds from her last pregnancy and decided that it was time to finally get serious about trying to lose the weight. After all, it had been seven years since her son had been born. Everything from the extreme diets to just plain skipping meals had been attempted in the last seven years. Nothing seemed to work. Dr. Warner was determined to take off those last stubborn ten pounds. She really didn't have a plan. She was going to eat less of everything and try to be busier in exercise and daily life. With Dr. Warner's having a busy medical practice, it was easy for her to skip meals. Often, there were night meetings after office hours, so it was hard to grab something nutritious to eat on the run between events. She decided a vegetarian diet sounded like a good idea (vegetarians always seemed so in control of their intake). Although nutrition education was only ten short days in medical school, she was pretty clear about what changes she needed to make in her diet to be a vegetarian—eliminate animal products.

Everything was going fairly well. The scales started to tip the other way, and gradually a few pounds started to melt off—until one day. That day started off as usual, but as the busy morning of seeing patients wore on, she noticed she was feeling very tired. In the late morning hours, while dictating notes to her tape recorder, the words just seemed harder to find.

During one of the last of the morning dictations, she noticed an overall body heaviness. When she tried to make a simple movement, or to take a step, it was as if the air was resisting her—as though all of her movements felt as if she were under water, and all forward motion was pushed back by a strong wall of water resistance.

She felt suddenly short of breath, sweaty, and thoughts and words were difficult to find. She leaned over her desk, sweating, gasping for air, heart pounding, shaking, feeling weak—trying to think clearly. Was this a heart attack, or a lung blood clot sucking the air from her chest?

Her nurse entered her office at this moment, and rushed to the doctor's side trying to assist. The doctor whispered to get a stat blood sugar. The doctor toppled in her chair while the nurse moved quickly to get a stat blood sugar. An unbelievable 32 mg/dl appeared on the blood sugar machine. It took three weeks of improved eating and adding animal protein products back into her diet before the doctor's blood sugar returned to a normal level.

Hypoglycemia: Low Blood Sugar

Extreme dieting can cause scenarios like the one described. All of the symptoms may not be as dramatic for you. Oftentimes, with extreme dieting (diets that eliminate all protein or all sugar), your blood sugar can drop, and you will feel light-headedness in the mid-morning or late afternoon. You can even faint during those times, due to low blood sugar. Other people will describe moodiness, hot flashes, dizziness, fatigue, weakness, shakiness, sinking feeling, or foggy thinking. These symptoms are often relieved by lying down or eating something.

The simple acts of lying down or eating something can relieve symptoms because blood sugar flow is restored to your brain. Your brain's fuel is blood sugar (or glucose). So, in order to maintain and restore its blood sugar flow to the brain, the brain will try everything—including making you faint so you are passed out flat on the floor—to make the bloodflow not have to work against the resistance of gravity to get to your brain.

Recently, one patient said that different friends has asked her to be a bridesmaid in their weddings, but every time she was in a wedding, she passed out at the alter. Upon examination, she realized that she had frequently tried to lose a few pounds before the wedding in order to look better in her dress, and this must have caused her blood sugar to drop low enough to make her pass out. Sure enough, a simple office test confirmed that she had hypoglycemia (or low blood sugar). If the earlier mentioned symptoms or situations sound familiar to you, you may want to ask your doctor for a three-hour glucose tolerance test. This is where you are fasting (no food for twelve hours) and a blood sugar is drawn for baseline. You are then given a sugary drink, and your blood sugar is drawn every hour for three hours thereafter. The result can be both enlightening and life-altering for you if you are found to have low blood sugar—hypoglycemia. Interestingly enough, our fear of meat and heavy proteins as being fatty and "bad" foods that should be avoided, may actually be triggering our blood sugar to dip low. This low blood sugar could be causing you to be shaky, weak, and foggy.

What is the treatment for hypoglycemia? Adding protein and complex carbohydrates (which are slowly digested and stored for a constant energy source) back into your diet to help sustain your body and keep you going. Proteins remain in your system and give you energy after the lighter or sugary foods, such as simple carbohydrates, have raced in and out of your system. The protein food you eat is the workhorse of your system; protein can get your body through your long day. While simple carbohydrates are better for giving you instant energy, they can't be relied upon for energy over the log haul. That is why eliminating protein while dieting for the "got to lose ten to twenty pounds before the 20-year high school reunion" leaves you feeling exhausted and starving. If the previously mentioned symptoms describe you, and you know your diet is frequently void of meats or fatty products, try choosing more foods that have more protein and complex carbohydrates. You may start to feel stronger and more energized throughout the day.

Diabetes: High Blood Sugar

What if you have the opposite? High blood sugar or diabetes? If you have what is now called Type 1 (formerly called juvenile diabetes) or Type 2 (formally called adult onset), the symptoms you feel may include the following: increased thirst, increased urination, burning with urination, numbness or tingling in hands or feet, slow-healing wounds, blurred vision, problems with sexual function, dizziness, flu-type symptoms of chronic achiness, recurrent abdominal pain, and sometimes even chronic diarrhea or nausea. Oftentimes, with increased blood sugar, you may notice you have more frequent infections or it takes you longer than you think it should to get over an infection. You may notice unexplained or recurrent vaginal yeast infections.

How do you figure out if your symptoms are due to diabetes? One of the newest practices is to have a blood sugar drawn two hours after a meal (non-fasting). This can sometimes help to diagnose you if you are borderline diabetic (blood sugar is higher than should be but close to normal). The standard blood sugar test is after an eight-hour fast. If your blood sugar is greater than 126 mg/dl on two separate days after fasting for eight hours, you are considered to be a diabetic. If your blood sugar non-fasting is greater than 200 mg/dl on two separate days, you are considered to be diabetic. If after two hours from eating your blood sugar is greater than 200 mg/dl during an oral glucose tolerance test, you are considered to be diabetic. One of the best ways to prevent and treat diabetes is by maintaining a normal weight and by choosing healthy foods. Although the American Diabetic Association does not currently endorse a particular diabetic diet, good choices are available through Weight Watchers or the Mediterranean Food Pyramid.

Your Personal Risk Assessment for Diabetes

	YES	NO
• Are you obese or 20 pounds overweight?	___	___
• Are you older than 45?	___	___
• Do you have a first degree relative with diabetes?	___	___
• Are you African American, Hispanic, Native American, Asian, or Pacific Islander?	___	___
• Did you have gestational diabetes or deliver a baby weighing greater than 9 pounds?	___	___
• Is your blood pressure typically greater than 140/90 m mHg?	___	___
• Is your HDL cholesterol less than 35?	___	___
• Is your triglyceride greater than 250 mg/dl?	___	___
• Have you had two separate fasting blood sugars greater than 126?	___	___

If you answered "yes" to several of the previous questions, then you may be at a higher risk for diabetes. You may need to have a blood sugar drawn by your doctor to screen for diabetes. It is very important that you are diagnosed and begin treatment of this silent killer. Think of diabetes as a glass of lemonade: you drank most (but not all) of the lemonade, and left the glass on the counter overnight. In the morning, the water had evaporated from the lemonade, and what remained was the crusty sugar remnants stuck to the glass. This is the same thing that happens to your body with diabetes. There is too much blood sugar in your arteries. You have too much sugar in your bloodstream and it gets stuck to your arteries, clogging the blood flow to your brain, heart, kidneys, eyes and nerves. For whatever reason, you don't have enough insulin in your body to carry the sugar into your organs and provide the organs with their needed sugar energy to fuel their jobs. Instead, the blood sugar remains in your blood vessels too long, clogging the major arteries to your vital organs. That is why diabetes is thought of as the silent destroyer, and can clog your major organs, such as your brain, eyes, nerves, kidneys, and heart. It is believed that 50 percent of the time if you are diagnosed with diabetes, you already have coronary artery disease. And, if you have diabetes, it is now considered a risk factor for coronary artery disease.

This all could be happening to you silently, and you may only have subtle symptoms like increased thirst or increased urination. Diabetes can seriously harm you. And if you are found to be diabetic, you need to work with your doctor to get you blood sugars to be normal (i.e. less than 110 mg/dl).

Diabetes is the number one cause of blindness in the United States, the number one cause of amputations, and the number one cause of kidney failure. If you are diabetic, you have four times the risk of having an amputation. You have four times the risk of having heart disease and stroke, and 75 percent of all diabetic people die of their heart disease. These things can be preventable with good control of your blood sugar.

At one time, it was believed that adult onset (Type 2) diabetes was not as significant or as dreadful as juvenile onset (Type 1) diabetes. Now, it is believed that they can both be as equally harmful to your body. Both types, regardless of whether you have Type 1 or Type 2, should be considered dangerous and destructive to your body. Both types need to be taken seriously by you. If diagnosed with either type, you should try to do lifestyle changes in an attempt to keep your blood sugar below 110 mg/dl. This way, your body may not be as harmed by this silent, sugar-clogging-artery-killer. If you are at high risk, or have symptoms of diabetes as mentioned earlier, or if you just have not been feeling yourself lately, you need to get a blood sugar drawn by your doctor. Controlling blood sugar may be your key to feeling better and living a longer, healthier life.

Health Tips for Blood Sugar:

- If two or more hours after a meal you start to feel shaky, light-headed, or weak, get a blood sugar drawn.
- If you are having increased thirst, increased urination, unexplained numbness or tingling in your hands or feet, slow healing wounds, blurred vision, problems with sexual function, and dizziness, get a blood sugar drawn.
- If you take your personal risk factors for diabetes quiz earlier in the chapter, and have several "yes" answers, you should get a blood sugar drawn.
- Diabetes is a silent killer. If you are diagnosed with diabetes, do everything you can to keep your blood sugar below 110 mg/dl.

Questions and Answers

Question #1: Can you have diabetes and hypoglycemia?
Answer: Yes, absolutely. Matter of fact, sometimes diabetics can have low blood sugars requiring a boost of sugar to bring their blood sugar back up to 65 mg/dl or greater.

Question #2: If you have hypoglycemia, can this lead to diabetes?
Answer: There is some thought that the pancreas (makes insulin) overworks itself producing insulin and eventually fizzles out and you become diabetic. It is best to have your blood sugars checked yearly if you are hypoglycemic. In addition, always eat a balanced and nutritious diet, exercise, and try to be near your ideal weight to help prevent diabetes.

Question #3: How often do you need blood sugars checked?
Answer: If you have risk factors, you should have yearly blood sugar screening done. If you are without risk factors and have no symptoms, have your blood sugar checked every three to five years.

Question #4: Is hypoglycemia connected to any other disorders?
Answer: In practice, I have noticed there seems to be some type of connection between hypoglycemia and thyroid disorders in women. So, it is a good idea, if you are not feeling quite right for several months, or are experiencing hypoglycemia and thyroid symptoms, to get a blood sugar and Thyroid Stimulating Hormone (TSH) drawn by your doctor.

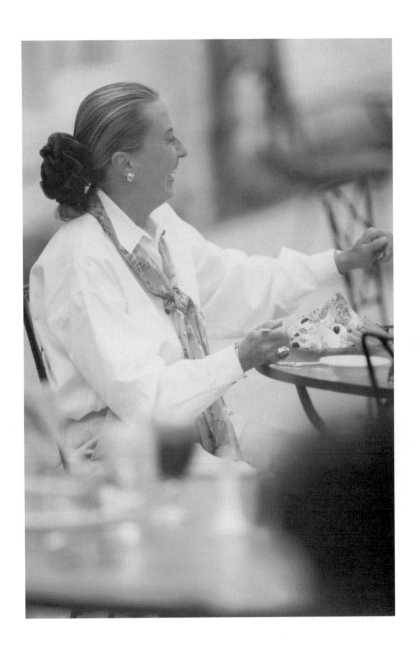

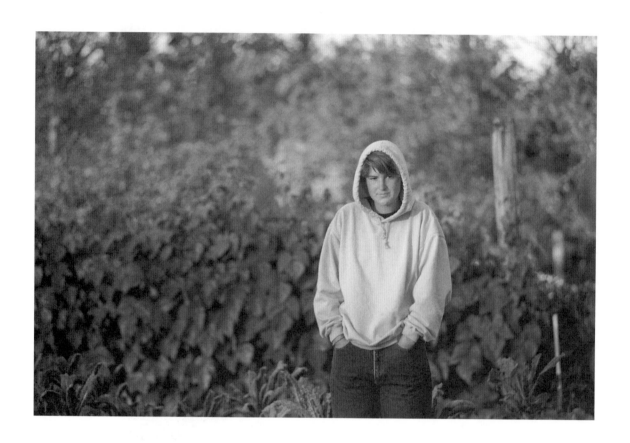

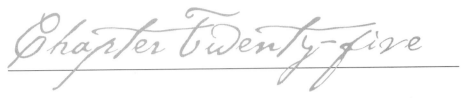

Chapter Twenty-five

You can't help the fact that you have a chemical imbalance. You can't wish, will, or want this imbalance away anymore than you can wish, will, or want a disease like diabetes away.

Chapter 25: Depression and Anxiety
Will the Real Me Please Stand Up?

Connie always seems to feel tired, lethargic, fatigued, run down, worn out, lacking energy and just plain exhausted. No matter how much sleep she gets, she never feels rested. She tries to go to bed earlier and sleep in later on weekends, but even if she sleeps longer, she still does not feel her energy is restored. On most days, Connie would prefer not to even get out of bed at all.

On the other hand, Tawny counted twelve times she awakened during the night last night. First she was hot and then she was cold. The covers were on, and off. Twice she ran for a bathroom break during the night. She couldn't seem to turn her brain off in order to fall asleep. Her list was long for the reasons why she could not sleep. After many restless nights, Tawny feels jumpy, wired, and easily irritated. And she drinks "way too much" caffeine to stay awake during the day.

In another instance, Lee can't seem to stop eating even when she should be full. She says she could eat five plates of food and still be hungry. She says she has "mental hunger." She knows her stomach is more than full but she keeps on eating because her spiritual side feels empty, and she is trying to fill that void and emptiness in her life by filling it with food. She knows food is a comfort to her and makes her feel loved and cared about, so she continues to eat to feed her empty soul. The scales tell her how wrong this lifestyle is, but to Lee it just does not seem to matter. What difference does it make, anyway, by adding a few more pounds to this already out-of-control situation, she thinks. Sometimes Lee feels it just doesn't matter what she looks like or what she weighs. Her being overweight is the punishment to herself for all the other failures in her life.

Tammy, on the other hand, can't seem to choke down even a morsel of food. The mere smell or sight of food makes her feel gaggy and nauseous. Even the normally tempting magazine and TV ads trying to entice her to eat leave her feeling nauseous. When she does try to eat a meal, Tammy finds herself only nibbling at her food and spends more time shoving her food around, rearranging and poking at her food in an attempt to make it appear to others she has eaten. Even when she does take some bites, the food seems to get stuck in her throat and it is hard to swallow.

Then there is Beth's story. Beth feels disconnected from her life and from herself. She was once a person who thoroughly enjoyed being with her friends and family, and she was always busy and on the go. She enjoyed being with her friends for dinner parties, meeting for lunch or coffee, or going to a movie together. Now, it seems she doesn't even want to leave her home. The simplest things make her eyes well up with tears. She no longer finds any pleasure in her hobbies like gardening. She can't seem to focus on anything, and her thoughts don't seem clear anymore. She is forgetful, misplacing items and not remembering what it was she walked into the next room to look for. Beth can barely function through today, let alone worry about tomorrow.

Do any of these sound familiar? You can have a few days in your life where the cylinders just aren't firing together for you and you feel "off balance." We all have great days full of joy and success and then some not-so-great days. If you find that your not-so-good days frequently outnumber your good days, you may be suffering from depression. Everyone in their lifetime will have at least two major depression episodes. The diagnosis of depression does not mean that you are weak in character and you should "toughen up." A diagnosis of depression does not mean you are "wacko." Every woman in her lifetime will go through some level of depression. It could be mild to severely disabling.

The more we understand depression, the more we realize it is a chemical imbalance in the brain's wiring with the chemicals that give a sense of peace and harmony. Sometimes depression is genetic. In depression there seems to be a lack of or depletion of neurotransmitters or brain chemical called serotonin, dopamine, or norepinephrine that causes a chemical imbalance and therefore depression. You can't help the fact that there is a chemical imbalance. You can't will, wish, or want this imbalance away anymore than you can will, wish, or want a disease like diabetes away. And just as diabetes requires a medicine, such as insulin or an oral agent to help restore blood sugar chemical balance, the neurotransmitter chemical imbalance you are experiencing may require medicine to restore your neurotransmitter chemical balance. And just like with diabetes, seeing a lifestyle nutritional counselor can help you have better control of your life; you may be light-years ahead in understanding what is going on with your body and mind if you work with a counselor. Take a minute right now to answer the survey on this page. Try to be very honest with yourself in answering the questions.

Your Personal Assessment for Depression*
(Symptoms felt most days for three or more weeks)

	YES	NO
• Do you feel irritable most of the time?	___	___
• Are you not able to concentrate?	___	___
• Do you have trouble enjoying your activities or interests?	___	___
• Have your sleep habits changed?	___	___
• Do you have more trouble making decisions?	___	___
• Have you changed weight unintentionally?	___	___
• Do you feel blue most of the time?	___	___
• Do you feel alone or want to be alone?	___	___
• Do you feel helpless or hopeless?	___	___
• Do you feel emotionless most of the time?	___	___
• Do you feel suicidal? (If you have suicide thoughts call your doctor now for help.)	___	___
• Do you feel tired despite getting enough sleep?	___	___
• Do you feel tearful most of the time?	___	___

*Adapted from the Zung Depression Scale

How did you do? If you answered "yes" to several of the questions, it is time to call your doctor and call a friend for help and support. You do not have to live like this any longer. Remember your survey score and read on. You may be suffering from depression and...

Anxiety

Linda is a worrier. She worries about everything, from what to have for dinner to what others think about her. She can never seem to relax. Even if she is sitting watching a television show she needs to have her legs crossed with her foot swinging and her hands fidgeting. Sometimes she notices her hands seem to even shake or tremble. Linda always feels tense and finds herself verbally snapping out at others, often inappropriately. Sometimes she feels her heart is beating too fast or has a choking sensation. Sometimes she even feels chest pain.* It is not uncommon for Linda to feel daily tension headaches.

Linda is suffering from anxiety. Just like depression, anxiety can be genetic and can be an imbalance. It is now felt that 50 percent of people suffering from depression also have anxiety and 50 percent of people suffering from anxiety have depression. Anxiety is a hypersensitivity to your body's wiring that can be exacerbated by your own thoughts. You are just more sensitive to your body's normal functioning. Your normal body function can seem exaggerated. With anxiety, normal things like heartbeat, muscle tension, body temperature, and breathing can all seem accelerated and exaggerated. Anxiety can be somewhat controlled with medicine, counseling, biofeedback, and reprogramming your brain's response to triggers by relaxation techniques. Take a minute right now to review the anxiety survey on the following page, and please be as honest with yourself as possible.

*All chest pain should be evaluated by a professional

Your Personal Assessment for Anxiety*

(Symptoms felt most days for three or more weeks; symptoms can occur even when not under stress)

	YES	NO
• Do you feel a choking sensation or have trouble swallowing?	___	___
• Do you have chest discomfort?	___	___
• Do you have shortness of breath?	___	___
• Does your heart race or skip a beat?	___	___
• Do your hands or body sweat easily?	___	___
• Do your hands get tingly?	___	___
• Do you feel detached or out-of-body sometimes?	___	___
• Do you feel faint or dizzy?	___	___
• Do you feel like you are losing control of body functions?	___	___
• Do you feel shaky or tremble?	___	___

*Adapted from the Buspar Anxiety Scale

Note: A form of anxiety is a panic attack which could have all of these symptoms, they would present and disappear in less then 15 minutes.

How did you do? If you found that you checked several "yes" answers and the symptoms seem present more often than not, you may have anxiety. You could benefit by calling your doctor for ideas on controlling your symptoms. Life can be better for you if you make the call and get back in control of your body.

You will go through phases in your life when you feel your emotions are in control of your mind, not your mind in control of your emotions. These phases can be a natural growing and maturing process. However, if you just can't seem to find "the real you," if you just don't feel like yourself week after week, or if you feel continually disconnected from your life and who you are, you may need to see your doctor. There may be a medical reason such as depression, anxiety, diabetes, thyroid disorder, or another type of medical imbalance that could be causing your symptoms. With the help of your doctor, you should be able to put your symptoms behind you and live your life more fully by enjoying your family, friends, hobbies, sports, work, and social life.

Your future potential is limited only by your own vision. With the help of your doctor, you can start to restore the balance of your spirit, mind, and body. The restored balance gives your life peace and harmony and allows you to be the best you can be doing the things you enjoy most in your life.

Questions and Answers

Question #1: It seems I mainly have symptoms of anxiety. What medicines are available for anxiety?
Answer: Common medications for anxiety:* Ativan, Paxil, Xanax, BuSpar, Serax, Zoloft, Effexor-XR, Valium, and Benzodiazepines.

Ativan has a longer half life, so it lasts in your system longer. It appears to last four to six hours in the blood stream. Ativan and Xanax are both medications that can be used prior to a stressful situation such as going to the dentist, giving a speech, or flying in a plane. Effexor-XR helps to decrease appetite so is a good choice if someone is depressed and is overweight. Paxil is one of the only ones approved for generalized anxiety disorder; Paxil can also treat panic and social anxiety disorder. Zoloft does a nice job with anxiety and depression and seems to be more weight and libido neutral. Ask your doctor to avoid the medicines that can cause weight gain and sleepiness. Non-medicine approaches include biofeedback, desensitization tricks, relaxation therapy, exercise, improving coping skills, counseling, and create a network of friends for support.

Question #2: It seems depression symptoms are what I mostly notice. The worst symptoms are avoiding social situations, snapping at others, and feeling blue. What are my medication choices for depression?
Answer: Common medications for depression:** Celexa, Elavil, Prozac/Sarafem, Desyrel, Pamelor, Remeron, Effexor XR, Paxil, Serzone, Zoloft, Wellbutrin SR, Sinequan.

Question #3: I have had only one depression episode after a stressful work situation. The depression seemed to resolve on its own. Can I expect to have another depression episode in my life?
Answer: It is important to remember that every single person will go through at least two major depressive episodes in her lifetime. This is not a sign of weakness nor of incompetence, you are simply not able to cope well with your life or with daily situations due to depression. This is merely a point in your life when your neurotransmitters are at a depleted level and, therefore, it makes it more difficult for you to function on your normally high level. Oftentimes, when you are hit with depression or anxiety, it is not something you can wish, will, or want away. It is a matter of a chemical imbalance that requires you to have your neurotransmitter stores replenished by the assistance of medicine. By going to your physician and stating you may need assistance with medicine for a brief period of time, you demonstrate inner strength and should be congratulated. **With the assistance and support of family and friends, counseling, and possibly medicine, you can start to fully enjoy your life again and live up to your full potential each and every moment. It is truly the journey that you should enjoy, not the destination. In order for you to allow yourself to enjoy each and every moment of your life, give yourself a chance to sparkle once again.**

*Other Benzodiazepines, Barbituates, and amitriptylines are available.
**Other Tricyclic antidepressants, amitriptylines, and monoamine oxidase inhibitors are available. Serotonin Reuptake Inhibitors seem to have fewer side effects than the old standard tricyclic anti-depressants. Choices include Celexa, Effexor XR, Luvox, Paxil, Zoloft, Serzone, Prozac/Sarafem (currently being used for premenstrual dysphoric disorder and PMS). Sarafem is a good choice to use 14 days before your period to control PMS symptoms. It may also be used daily. Prozac has one pill that you can take once weekly (which is great for convenience and compliance). Zoloft is a good choice for anxiety, obsessive compulsion and depression; Zoloft seems to have less effect on libido and weight than some. Zyprexa, formerly used for acute manic of bipolar, is now being used for more complicated anxiety/depression. Remeron is great for insomnia and decreased appetite. Wellbutrin works well for depression. It also helps decrease desire for nicotine, assisting with smoking cessation. It should be avoided by anyone with a seizure history. It also seems to be more weight neutral and in some cases actually may increase libido. Zoloft is the number one selling antidepressant. Non-medicine approaches include biofeedback, goal-setting, exercise, improving coping skills, counseling, hobbies and crafts, reconnecting a network of friends for activities and support.

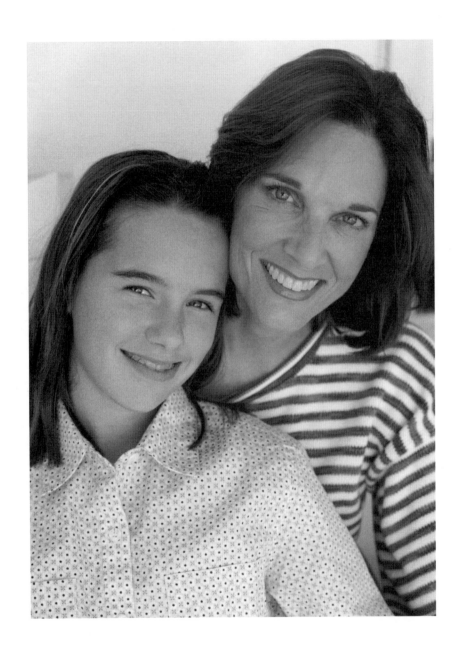

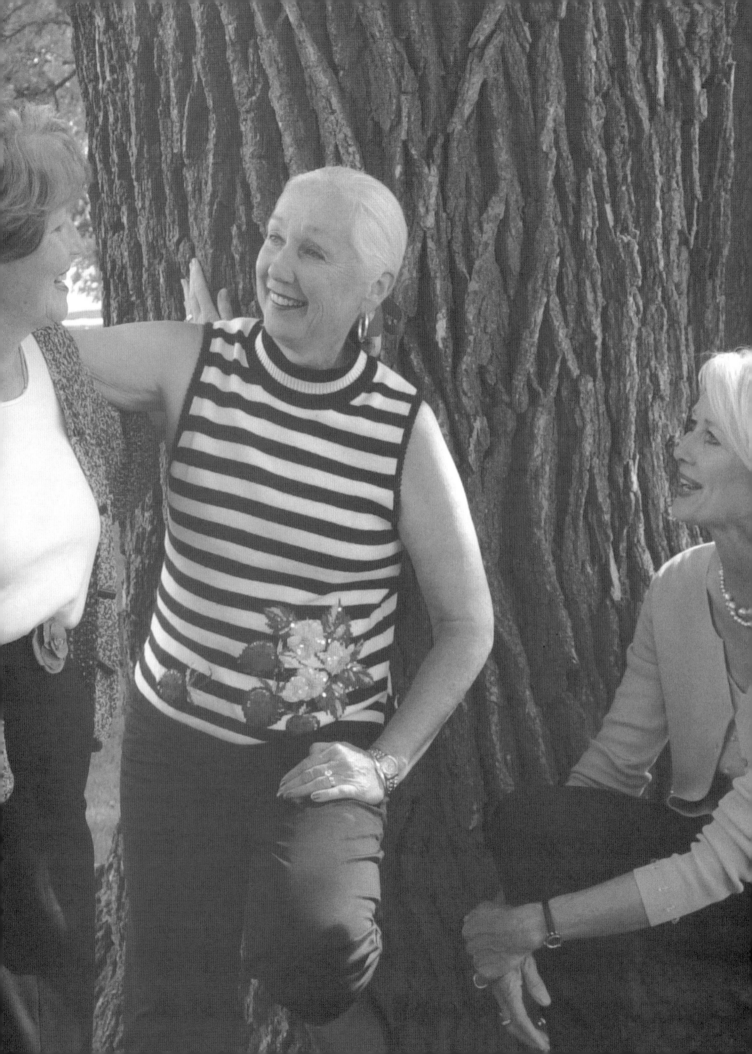

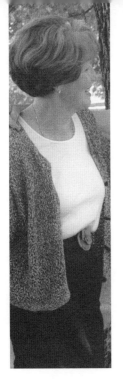

Personal Style

Your clothing should be your second skin. Your clothing should be a reflection of you and should be your personal statement. Your clothes should allow you to express yourself and give you complete freedom from ever having to think about what you are wearing.

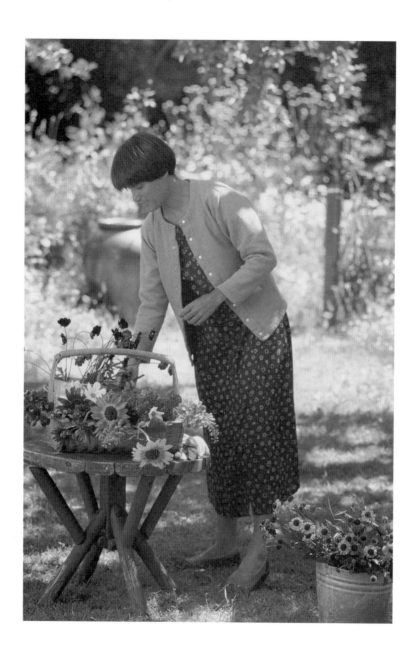

No longer do you have to follow trends, fads, or other people's senses of style. Create your own image and define your own look. Who knows? You may even start a trend of your own!

Chapter 26: Finding Your Personal Style The Secret to Fashion

One of the gifts of aging is being able to find a sense of style and that expresses you are and who you have evolved into. This allows you the confidence to be you. Your clothes should be a reflection of who you are or who you want to be. Don't try to copy someone else's sense of style from a magazine or a friend that you admire. Strike your own personal fashion pose using your own unique style. Be true to yourself and let yourself shine by selecting styles of clothing that enhance your body and personality. It is okay to be you. Communicate through your clothes in order to make a personal statement. **The beauty of discovering your own personal style is that there are no fashion rules; you rule your own personal fashion statement! If it feels right for you, it is right. No longer do you have to follow trends, fads, or other people's senses of style. Create your own image and define your own look. If a camel hair, double-breasted jacket, popular in the 1970s defines you and makes you feel powerful and elegant, let it be your signature jacket and wear it with a flare. Who knows? You may even start a trend of your own!**

The secret to style is to put on the garment and then close your eyes and forget for a moment what the garment looks like. Probe all your senses to see how the garment makes you feel when you wear it. If the garment makes you feel good, the way you want to feel, you own it. It's yours. It defines who you are and you should wear it with pizzazz. Go through your closet and hold or try on each item and think about how it makes you feel. If it makes you feel good and helps you to create a style statement of what you want to say, keep it and enjoy it. If a garment does not make you feel good for whatever reason, give it up. Release it from your sentimental grip. You don't want to own something that isn't right or doesn't allow you to feel good. If this garment owns you and competes with your ability to enjoy your day, or this garment is selfishly distracting your attention every time you wear it (not fitting correctly, binding you, or not being a flattering color), then it controls you and distracts your attention, not allowing you to be the one in control. You want to choose clothing that is in sync with you and your personal sense of style so when you wear it you can forget about it and enjoy your day.

It has been said that our clothing should be our "second skin." Your clothing should be a reflection of you and should be your personal statement. Your clothes should allow you to express yourself and give you complete freedom from ever having to think about what you are wearing. They should fit, flatter, and make you feel confident enough that you can completely forget about yourself and your clothing and focus on the moment of your life that you are experiencing.

Do you have a favorite, comfy uniform that you put on the minute you enter the sanctuary of your own home? An outfit that bathes you with coziness and makes you feel wrapped in total acceptance as if you were in comfortable, protective arms? You might want to rethink that outfit. If that same outfit leaves you feeling like you want to dive under the bed or grab a jacket to cover yourself up if the doorbell should ring unexpectedly, chances are you could find an outfit that is more flattering but still comfortable.

My favorite home outfit used to be a discarded, discolored shirt of my brother's. It was a red, black, and white torn and threadbare plaid flannel. The shirt topped off dingy, gold sweat pants that had shrunk too short. The sweatpants were missing the draw string, so the waist was gathered together into a wad clasped with a giant safety pin. Completing the ensemble were poorly fitting, dingy-white athletic socks. This was my comfy home outfit.

Finally, one day it struck me that I would spend one hour primping, polishing, perfuming, glossing, moussing, and dressing to make a one-second great impression on a complete stranger, but would only spend one second on how I looked when I got back to the comforts of home for myself or for the important people who shared my home. After I came to the realization that I needed to feel good about myself and my appearance in the comforts of my home, I decided to start wearing things that were just as comfortable but a tad easier on the eye than my lovely gold sweat pants. Just in case an unexpected guest happened to stop by, I would not have to be embarrassed by my appearance and hide behind the door, but would have on an outfit that was comfortable and gave me enough confidence that I would not have to think about my appearance and just be able to focus my attention on the guest.

Also, go through your underwear drawer and see if you can honestly say that your undergarments are in good working order, and they make you feel comfortable and confident. If they do, keep them. But, if you look at that garment and say, "I hope no one ever knows I am wearing this worn-out thing," then replace it. Purchase something that makes you feel sassy, special, and attractive—you deserve it!

Tips for Style

- Buy a clothing items that allows you to feel good about yourself.
- Forget trends, fads, or other people's styles. Find clothing that expresses the unique you.
- Don't hold yourself hostage to your own previous self-image. If you have to wear navy suits Monday through Friday, do "styling" on the evenings and weekends to set your self-expression free.
- Try something new like thong underwear. Maybe you will surprise yourself and discover something new that is really "you."
- What color is right for you? You will know because you feel good when you wear it. Everyone seems to compliment you on it and you don't even seem to need to wear makeup when you have that color on.
- Let your style reflect you. Wear what makes you feel good and helps you to communicate how you feel about yourself.
- In your fashion-show runway of life, you can choose to strike any pose you want to by the clothing that you choose to wear. It is your show. Be the star and let yourself shine by choosing clothes that let you be your own unique self.
- Have fun, smile, and enjoy yourself no matter what you are wearing. Style starts on the inside with your self-contentment and personal harmony. Your clothing is only an accessory of outward expression to your inner spirit and sense of self.

The secret to personal style and color of clothes that you select is how they make you feel. It has almost nothing to do with the look. Your style is defined by how the clothes make you feel. If the outfit lets you feel slinky, sassy, or sophisticated, then you will look and act slinky, sassy, or sophisticated in it. That is the secret to style. Style starts with you and how you feel about yourself. This feeling will be the image you are expressing through your clothes. You choose the self-image that you want to express by the ensemble in which you choose to present yourself.

In selecting clothes, the number one most important person to please is yourself. Choose clothing that makes you feel how you want to feel, and select the colors that create a good feeling or mood when you wear them. You don't have to follow books, charts, or graphs to try and figure out what clothing style and colors are right for you. You'll know it when you feel it. When you feel good, you look good. Only then have you discovered your personal style. When you choose your clothing—not by how they make you look but how they make you feel—you will always choose the outfit, color, and style that is just right for you.

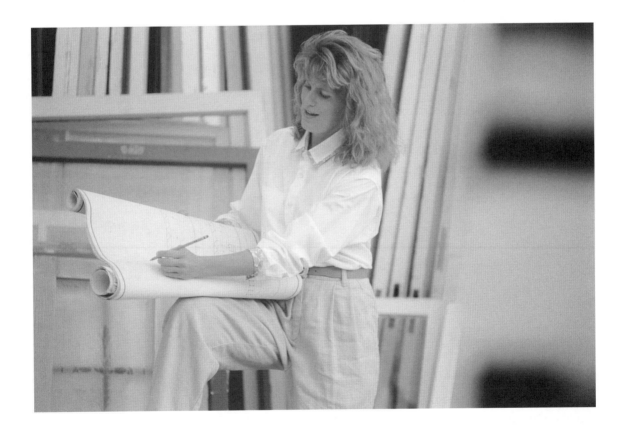

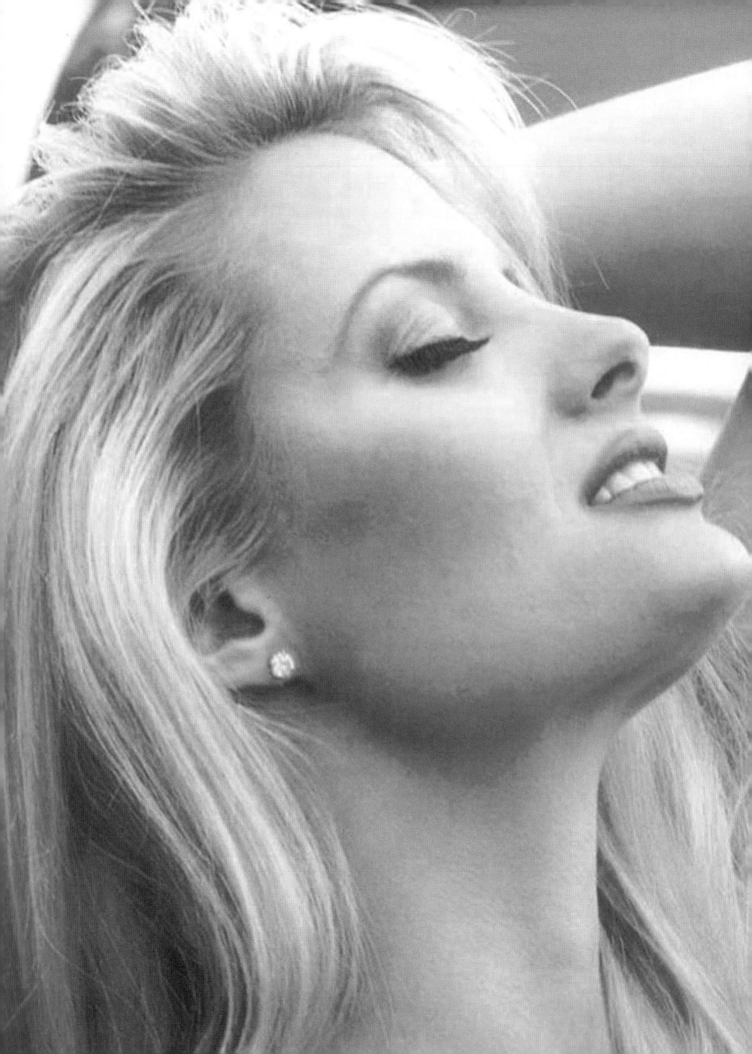

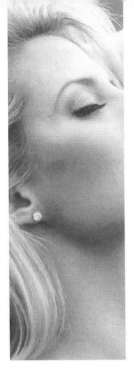

Sparkle

A Fresh Start to a New You

Wake up in the morning and know that you are beautiful. This is your day. Rejoice and rejuvenate and know this is going to be a great day for you. Think three positive thoughts to start your day. Do this every morning.

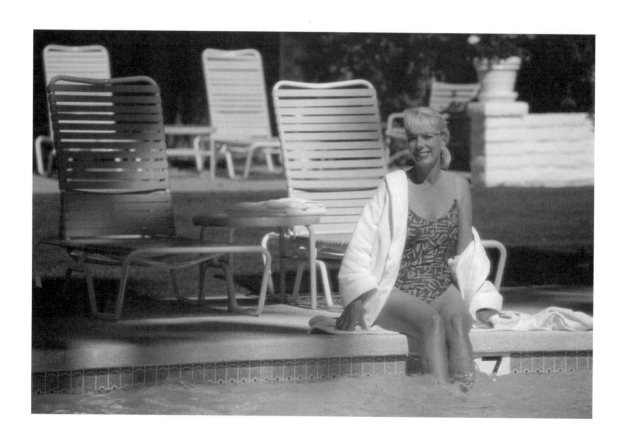

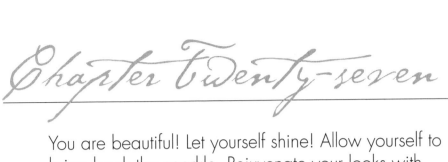

Chapter Twenty-seven

You are beautiful! Let yourself shine! Allow yourself to bring back the sparkle. Rejuvenate your looks with skincare, a new hairdo, and a splash of makeup that is just right for you. You are a diamond just waiting to be polished in order to sparkle with inner and outer beauty.

Chapter 27: Sparkle
A Fresh Start to a New You

Tammy is double-take beautiful. Tammy and her business partner Anne own an upscale interior decorating salon. Anne says that when they go on business trips together that men's heads swivel to get a second look at this gorgeous woman walking through the show room. Tammy is 45 years of age and has timeless good looks, a sculptured face, and impressive eyes.

During her physical, Tammy mentioned she would like to get a referral to a plastic surgeon to see what could be done about the small wrinkle lines around her mouth area. Having to stand up from my exam chair and walk to within a few feet of Tammy in order to see the almost microscopic lines to which she was referring, I agreed to send her to see a plastic surgeon. I was totally amazed at the letter we received back from the plastic surgeon.

Evidently, in addition to the fine mouth wrinkles, Tammy and the plastic surgeon also discussed the aging around her eyes and lower face. The plastic surgeon had recommended to start off with a brow-lifting, upper and lower blepharoplasty (eyelid "lift" surgery), a face "lift" underneath the chin, jaw liposuction, lip fat grafts—and to top everything off—a full-face chemical peel to diminish her facial creases. And here we had all thought that Tammy was gorgeous!

Fortunately, Tammy realized that beauty starts from the inside and radiates to the outside with a healthy, happy spirit. Tammy chose to first make a few lifestyle changes before considering going through surgery. She is going to stop the occasional cigarette smoking, start eating more fruits and vegetables and less fast and convenient foods, incorporate exercise into her day, and start using rejuvenating lotions and creams.

Beauty starts from within, with your personal and mental thoughts about yourself and your overall self-image. You have to first learn to like and accept yourself for what and who you are. You have to first like yourself and then you can highlight, enhance, and accentuate your outside features with the right skin care, haircut, and makeup. All the plastic surgery and makeup that your money can buy still cannot—and will not—change a discontented heart and spirit. First, start to see the beauty that is inside of you.

The first thing you need to do to cleanse your spirit is to look into the mirror and see yourself for the special person you are and your own natural beauty. It is okay to love and respect yourself—just don't be in love with yourself. If you feel better about yourself, you will radiate and glow outwardly. The better you feel about yourself, then the more you can love others and live up to your potential and fulfill your goals. You must allow yourself to reach this level of confidence.

When you reach the level where you can feel good about yourself, you can then forget about yourself and focus on others!

You are beautiful! Let yourself shine! Allow yourself to bring back the sparkle. Rejuvenate your looks with skincare, a new hairdo, and a splash of makeup that is just right for you. You are a diamond waiting to be polished in order to sparkle with inner and outer beauty. True beauty allows you to feel great about yourself from the inside to the outside. Let yourself sparkle!

How your skin appears can affect how you see yourself as a person. When your skin is soft, supple, and has minimal wrinkles, you radiate a glow to others; it is as if you have defied the aging process.

In order to have beautiful skin, you need to understand your basic skin structures. The dermis is the deepest layer of your skin and has all the elastic fibers and collagen that support your skin and make it appear toned and firm. With aging, the elastic fibers and collagen support start to give way. Creases, wrinkles, and drooping occur around your eyes, forehead, and lip area.

The top visible layer is the epidermis. The epidermis provides color, protection from the environment, and moisture. As the skin ages, it can become dry, thin, shiny, wrinkled, pale or blotchy in color, and can develop skin spots. As the skin ages, it also loses its moisture and elasticity. Acne and age spots can form. Of course, sun exposure can accelerate any aging process to your skin. Staying out of the sun and using protective lotions and clothing may help prevent sun damage to your skin. On the following page are a few special beauty secrets to help you feel beautiful from the inside to the outside.

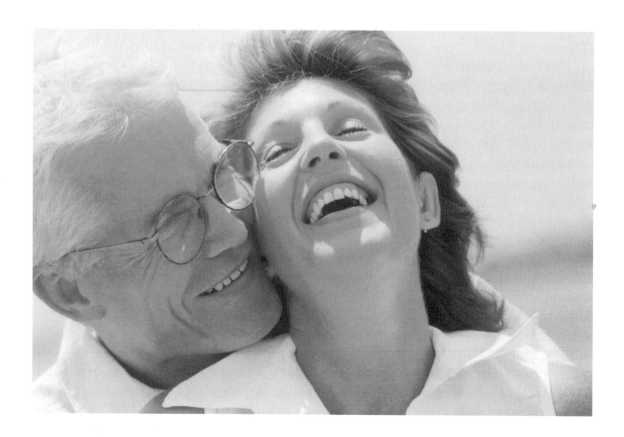

A Fresh Start for a New You!

Morning Secrets:

Rejuvenate

Wake up in the morning and know that you are beautiful. This is your day. Rejoice and rejuvenate and know this is going to be a great day for you. Think three positive thoughts to start your day. Do this every morning.

Energize

Energize and empower yourself with inner and outer strength by doing a rejuvenating exercise routine each day. Exercise gets your heart pumping and blood to your tissues. Exercise tones your muscles, making you feel fit and confident. It also helps prevent cancers, heart disease, and diabetes. Inches will melt away and you will feel great and in control.

Fortify

Fortify your energy with a healthy breakfast to keep your engine humming all day long. Get eight hours of sleep, eat a balanced diet, and don't smoke. Add a multivitamin and take calcium (1200 mg per day) for extra protection. Remember: drinking 64 ounces of water a day moisturizes your skin.

Sparkle: Beauty secrets for the face and neck area

Morning secrets to maintain and restore daily your natural skin beauty:

Cleanse

Splash water and use a cosmetic cleanser or mild bar of soap to clean your face and neck using your hands only. Blot dry with a cotton towel. Blotting prevents wrinkles.

Exfoliate

Use an exfoliative product to wash away old skin cells to allow young, fresh, rejuvenated skin to appear. Exfoliate one to three times a week to keep your skin looking its best. Add a facial oil every other day if your skin becomes too dry.

Moisturize

Get the youthful glow back by adding a moisturizer to your skin. Gently apply lotion around the eye area, being careful not to put lotion just below your eye, or just above the eye on the lid area—these areas will absorb the lotion and the result will be puffiness. Gently pat until absorbed. Choose a foundation that has a moisturizer for extra moisture. Remember to select products that have SPF for protection from the sun.

Specialty Creams

Prevent wrinkles and protect skin from sun, pollutants, smog, and free radicals with anti-aging face and eye creams. Select products that have vitamin A and C derivatives that help to diminish fine lines. Retinol, alpha hydroxy acid, and beta hydroxy acids are names to look for on the label.*

Nighttime Secrets to help you look forever young; choose your favorite brands that work the best for you:

Eye makeup removal

Any eye makeup remover helps gently remove eye makeup without stretching and causing wrinkles to the delicate skin around your eyes.

Cleanse

Splash water and use a cosmetic cleanser or mild bar of soap to clean your face and neck using your hands only. Blot dry with a cotton towel. Blotting prevents wrinkles.

Tone

A toner helps clarify your skin by removing flaky, loose skin cells. It removes blotchy or spotty areas. A toner can leave your skin smoother, cleaner, and more toned.

Moisturize

A moisturizer restores your skin's resistance and resilience while making it supple, soft, and smooth. A moisturizer restores your youthful glow. Use only pin-dot amounts of moisturizer around the eye area to preven puffiness. Use specialty creams such as anti-aging or eye creams to protect skin and prevent aging.

*Retinoicacid derivative products (Retin-A, Renova) are available by prescription. Retinol is in over-the-counter products.

Body: Skin-firming lotions and cellulite creams

Cellulite can not be rubbed away with a cream, Cellulite is stored fat under the skin. The only way to remove cellulite is by toning up and maintaining a healthy weight. However, there are creams available that temporarily tighten the skin so you see less dimpling of the cellulite on the skin surface.

Prevention Treatment of Aging Skin and Wrinkles

- Avoid the direct sun exposure.
- Use SPF makeup, sunscreen, visors, and hats.
- Drink 64 ounces of water a day, sleep eight hours a night, don't smoke, exercise, and eat a well-balanced diet.
- Alpha hydroxy acids, beta hydroxy acids, retinol, and other products containing vitamin A and C seem to help diminish fine lines. (Look for these anti-wrinkle ingredients on the label of products you buy.)

Tricks of the Trade:

A makeup brush is an absolute must for any natural-appearing beauty; it separates those with good looks from those that appear to be a natural beauty. With your brush, blend, blend, blend and when you think you have blended enough blend some more. You need two brushes. One larger brush to use over the cheek and entire face area to smooth makeup lines and to blend colors. A smaller brush is used to blend eye shadows and eye creams.

Finishing Touches:
Concealers

We all have areas we would like to accentuate or to conceal. There are several choices of concealers:
- Green concealer: covers red, ruddy blemishes and spider veins
- Yellow: conceals dark circles
- Purple: is excellent for highlighting your best features, like high cheek bones

Foundation

Add a smooth and silky finish only where you need it. Look for foundations that have a moisturizer and SPF protection.

Your Other Choices: Done by a Professional

Facial Masks and/or Facial Massages
- Chemical peel: uses a chemical to remove the top layers of the skins epidermis to reveal softer and smoother skin
- Microdermabrasion: uses a chemical product that is blown with force on the skin and then removed. Leaves the skin feeling fresh, soft, and smooth
- Dermabrasion: uses scraping to remove the top layers of the skin's epidermis. The refinishing leaves the skin smoother and softer
- Laser: uses the laser's heat to remove the top layers of the skin's epidermis and wrinkles. Helps to remove the blotchy or spotty skin colors and smooth out thickened areas. Works well for lip, eye, and forehead areas
- Injection Choices:

   Microliposuction: body fat is injected to lip, nose, or chin area

   Collagen, silicone, or Gore-Tex ™ injectables

   Botulinum toxin (botox): an FDA approved to treat wrinkles

Dazzle: Choosing the perfect color pallets for you

Your Eyes:
- Blue Eyes: use eye shadows that are earth tone, brown, beiges and creams, mauves, some violets to grays, charcoal, and medium gray
- Green Eyes: choose eye shadows with earth tones, mauves, purples and pinks
- Brown Eyes: choose eye shadows with pinks, earth tones, bright purples, bright blues, or vivid colors

Your Cheeks:
- Fair: choose blush colors that are light pinks, beiges, or corals
- Medium skin: select blush colors that are deep rose, mauves, or browns
- Olive: select from deeper mauves, browns, or roses

Your Lips:
- Thin to appear Fuller: use a lip liner outside the natural lip line and fill in with a similar colored lipstick
- Full to appear thin: use a lip liner inside the natural lip line and use a similar colored lipstick

Lip color choices:
- Fair skin tone: light pinks, mauves, peaches, coral, or nudes
- Medium skin tone: rose, reds, light browns, earth tones, or nudes
- Olive to dark skin tone: deeper reds, plums, fuchsia, or roses

Sparkle

It feels good to have a fresh start for a new you. You are rejuvenated, energized, fortified, and you are sparkling. You look magnificent. Let yourself shine with beauty from the inside to the outside. There is nothing you can't accomplish. You are reenergized and empowered. Go out and make a difference in your life and in the lives of those whom you touch.

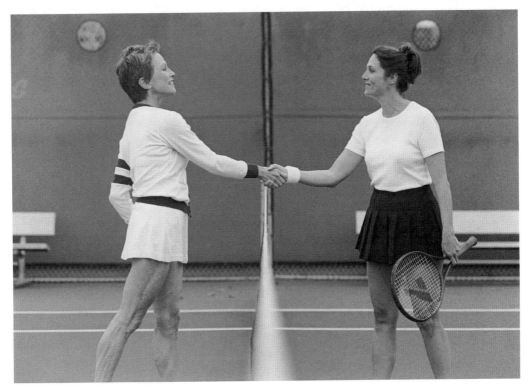

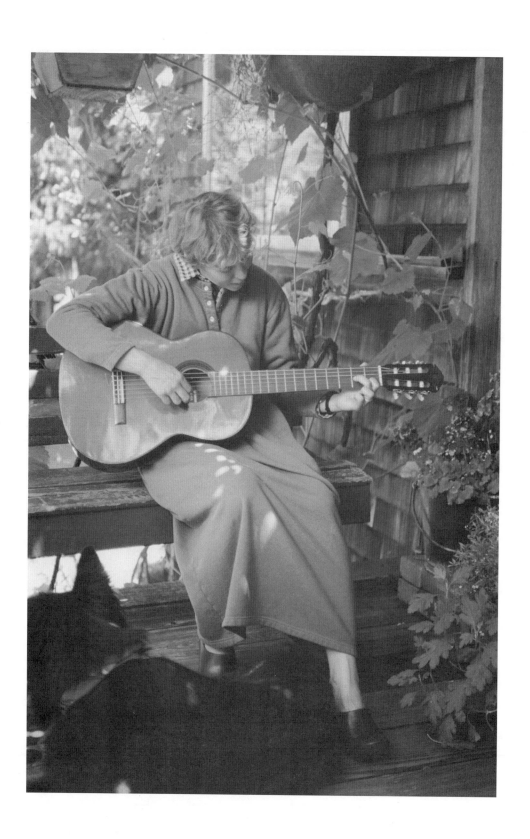

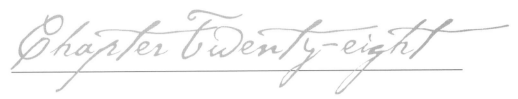

Chapter Twenty-eight

Release your mind and free yourself from the mental chains that hold you down and keep you from evolving and acquiring new hobbies, activities, and interests. You can do and become anything you can imagine.

Chapter 28: Changing the Face of Beauty Balancing Spirit, Mind, and Body

Spirit: You are beautiful, right now just as you are—right where you are in your life's journey. With aging comes the power of expression. You have finally arrived at a point in your life when you (hopefully) have some freedom of choice in who you are and how you want to live. You have the opportunity to change those things about yourself and your life that may be holding you hostage to the past. You can now control your decisions regarding what matters most to you. You can control your thoughts of who you are and your own self-image. No longer do you have friends, classmates, or co-workers who define and pigeonhole you. You are free to choose who you are and how you want to present yourself to the world. Now is the time to dare to imagine yourself as better. These are the best years of your life, right now. Claim your age. Embrace your age. Own your age. Reclaim yourself. Stop comparing yourself to a 21-year-old in a thong bikini who has never had children. You don't really want to go back there in those uncertain, insecure, financially-dependent-on-your-parent times, do you?

Now is the time to celebrate your arrival to the full spectrum of the evolving you—in all your dazzling glory. Don't think of beauty as it was defined for you at age twenty. Think of a new definition of beauty that evolves with you—the changing face of beauty. This changing face of beauty warmly embraces your age and cherishes your youth—as you will never be younger than you are right now, at this very moment. With claiming every year of your life, you can allow yourself the opportunity to celebrate and express yourself and your beauty right now—just where you are, just as you are at this moment in time.

Beauty does not come from a facelift or expensive clothing. Beauty radiates to the outside from your inner spirit from you being happy and satisfied with who you are. One of the gifts of aging is having less of a fear of other people's opinions. You have the power to create your own self image by the thoughts you have of yourself. You can expect more of yourself now, but you have to believe in yourself and believe that you—and you, alone—are able to achieve peace, harmony, and balance within your own spirit, mind, and body. When you look in the mirror at yourself, who do you see? Your impression of your own reflection is the image you are giving to others through your facial expressions and body language. The outward appearance is driven by your own self image. Being your age and beyond can be hot! You can be hot! You have to have the self-confidence that only age can bring to your perspective of who and what you are. Desire to be your best right now, and enjoy your incredible journey.

Tips for Enhancing Your Spirit:

- Upon awakening, think three happy thoughts about your life.
- Think three positive thoughts about yourself.
- Say three positive things out loud today.
- Call, write, e-mail, or visit a family member or friend today.
- Smile and laugh today.
- Go out of your way to give someone joy today.
- Take a bubble bath.
- Get a massage.
- Listen to your favorite CD.
- See a movie with a friend.
- Send someone flowers.
- Look in the mirror and smile at who you see.
- Learn to love who you are.
- Be happy with your life and who you are right now—at this moment.

Mind: When you look into the mirror, who do you see? Are you surprised that the youthful, eager, unstressed face of a woman you expect to see has been replaced with a face of a woman who is a wife, mother, grandmother, volunteer, chauffeur, counselor, and homemaker? Do you even recognize yourself in your own reflection? Are you so busy being busy that you have lost who you are and why you exist? Have you pushed the hold button on your life and placed your dreams, goals, and ambitions into a time capsule as you frantically race through your life caring for everyone else but yourself?

This is the way it was meant to be, isn't it? In your youth, you fantasized you would be lucky enough to have a rich and fulfilling family life and career. So why aren't you vibrantly flourishing? Why aren't you leaping with boundless energy and why are you not happy? Why, instead, are you exhausted and just barely making it through your stressful day's events? Of course, there is no time for you. That would be selfish and unjustified. After all, there is always another load of laundry you could be doing. This is the way it is supposed to be, and you had better keep going and not stop for a second because everyone in your world is depending on you! Right? You couldn't be more wrong. Rethink and redefine your role.

One of my mentors, who has been practicing medicine for 35 years, quietly watched as I went through my day bolting from one activity to another, as if being paced by a stopwatch. He came up to me one day, after watching this frantic display of activity, and said he wanted to talk to me. He sat me down in my office and looked at me—with eyes that showed years of wisdom—and said, "Who should be the most important person in your life?"

Without hesitation, I said, "God."

He said, "That's a given, who's next?"

I quickly and dutifully said, "My husband." His intensity sharpened, and he patiently asked me again, "Who should be the most important person in your life?" Now, I was searching my mind. What was he looking for?

"My kids," I blurted out, anxiously waiting to see his approving nod. Instead, I saw his eyes look disappointed and his head slowly shake "no." Now, I was guessing and looking for approval as I spurted out, "Okay, my parents." That had to be it. I should have thought of it earlier. I hoped that answer would please my mentor.

Slowly, he leaned forward and barely above a whisper said, "You." Could I have heard him right? How could it be me? First, that would be incredibly selfish and self-centered to even think of myself first, and second, I would actually have to put on hold being a wife, mother, daughter, and sister to have time to make myself number one.

"Me?" I blurted out.

"Yes, you," he said. "You need to be number one on your priority list because all of these other people are depending on you to be the very best wife, mother, daughter, and sister that you can be. If you are not the very best person you are capable of being, and happy with what and who you are, nothing else in your life will click. You don't have time *not* to make yourself number one. A lot of people are depending on you to be healthy in spirit, mind, and body; so you can be there whole and complete to make their world go round."

My mentor was right. In your busy world of many roles, your time to reclaim who you are is **now**. This very moment in your life is a wonderful chance to rediscover who you are and reclaim your visions, dreams, and aspirations. Now is the time to strengthen and enhance your mind. Your mind craves sensory input through the arts that add color and life to your world. Your mind needs enrichment through indulging yourself in a mental activity. Your mind needs challenges to strive to a new level of wisdom. If you are able to give your mind a few moments of your time each day, your mind will reward you by feeling refreshed, restored, and rejuvenated. Don't you think you have the time to indulge yourself and rediscover and reclaim you and who you are?

At a motivational lecture, Zig Ziglar said, "You can change yourself by what goes into your mind and body. We all have the same 24 hours. There is no such thing as lack of time. Just lack of direction. Plan, prepare, and expect to win. It is not what happened to you, but how you handled it. In order to win at life, you need to rise above your limits both real and imaginary. In other words, you need to visualize yourself as successful, well-balanced, and healthy. Change your current picture of yourself and visualize yourself as already 'there' and then it is your job to maintain that success. Claim your good qualities."

It is not where you started, or when you started, but where you end up. You are already born with all the skills and qualities you will ever need to find harmony and balance between your spirit, mind, and body; it is your new vision of yourself that will allow you to enhance and enrich those skills and qualities. Right now, inside of you, is the person you are searching for. Right now is a wonderfully opportune time to look in the mirror and see a new view of you. The beautiful gift of aging is that you are continually evolving every day.

Today is your chance for a new opportunity to try something new and different. Stop setting mental self-imposed limits and boundaries on your life. Release your mind and free yourself from the mental chains that hold you down and keep you from evolving and acquiring new hobbies, activities, and interests. You can do and become anything you can imagine. You are only limited by your own vision. Look into the mirror and see a new and improved reflection of yourself. There is no such thing as being too old to make a change to become who you want to be. Redefine yourself and reclaim yourself. Your future is only limited by your own imagination.

Now it is your turn and your time. Today is your day to be the best you can be. The rich and beautiful benefits of enriching yourself will cascade over your world and into all the lives you touch. Allow time for yourself to refresh, restore, and rejuvenate your mind.

Tips for Enhancing Your Mind:

- Enjoy a hobby, art, or music today.
- Read, write, play a game, watch a movie, or do some type of mental exercise today.
- Enable yourself to get seven to eight hours of restorative sleep tonight.
- Spend 15 minutes for you today, indulging in an activity that refreshes, restores, and rejuvenates you.
- Do not smoke or use any type of drug that will alter your ability to restore and rejuvenate your mind.
- Take a painting class.
- Buy a new CD.
- Visit an art center.
- Play a television game along with the contestants.
- Rent a favorite movie.
- Read a romantic novel.
- Savor the moment you are in with your current surroundings and environment.
- Take a correspondence class on the Internet.

Body: Aging is not the beginning of the end, and the way your life has been isn't the way it always has to be in the future. Now is a second chance for a new beginning and for becoming a new and improved you, capable of feeling strong, healthy, and energized ready for your fantastic future. The best is yet to come.

In his article "Use it or Lose it," Walter Bortz, M.D., states, "What we once considered to be marks of aging, we now know are the results of disease or disuse." Dr. Bortz also states, "If you make a list of all of the changes in the human body that are ascribed to aging—changes in muscle, bones, brain, cholesterol, blood pressure, sleep habits, sexual performance, psychologic inventory, and so forth—and compile a similar list of changes due to physical activity, you will notice a striking similarity between the two lists...Many of the bodily changes we always ascribed to the normal aging process are, in fact, caused by disuse." In other words, as you age, it is somewhat your choice if you want to become lethargic, shriveled, and fragile with a low muscle mass due to disuse, thereby giving up your freedom and independence and getting stuck in a nursing home.

You are not a victim of your own body, and the world is not holding you hostage to your formal lifestyle habits. Sometimes it does seem as though you frantically try to follow your dream of an improved and better lifestyle, only to be sabotaged by food commercials, parties, and life's events. You must give yourself permission to like yourself enough to succeed and be your best. You, alone, have the choice to control your future destiny. Choose to be healthy now and in your future by making daily lifestyle choices that keep you focused on being your best. Do you want to be 70 years of age in a nursing home, bound to a geriatric chair, being spoon-fed because when you were younger you made choices to indulge in your desires? The fat, sugar, and lack of physical activity caused the increased cholesterol that clogged your arteries, and caused a major stroke that accounts for your merely surviving your time in a nursing home. Instead, do you want to make simple lifestyle choices today that allow you to be rewarded with the freedom to be energized, active, and to live a robust future? So, at age 70, you will be deciding whether to hike or bike your way up a mountain rather than deciding whether to eat Jell-O or pureed custard through a straw at the nursing home.

Do not be paralyzed with the fear of failure, locking yourself into old habits of food cravings and eating for comfort. This will not allow you to be a better you. In order to get to where you need to go, you will need to take a step in a different direction. One step in any direction is better than standing still locked in your self-imposed, previous habits that keep you paralyzed in your present. One little step towards eating healthy is a giant step taken toward your goals and dreams. By taking one little step, you are one step closer to being where you want to be. Stop supersizing your servings to fill your life's voids and start maximizing a vision of a new and improved you. To begin, avoid your old, bad habits. Don't buy the chips that will sit on your shelf, causing the visual stimulation to eat them. It is best to just never start eating the chips. If you don't start eating the chips, you don't have to decide when to stop.

Tips for Enhancing Your Body:
- Eat more vegetables and fruit today.
- Exercise 30 minutes today.
- Do toning activities today.
- Do not overeat today.
- Drink 64 ounces of water today.
- Think of safety and prevention in all that you do today.
- Rethink what sounds tasty.
- Fill the voids in your soul with music, and life, not food.
- Exercise for the 30 minutes instead of reading the paper.
- Take the stairs, park further from work today.
- View a three-pound weight as your toning friend.
- Do not eat more than one cup serving size of any food today.
- Reach for a glass of water instead of pop, coffee, or tea today.
- Wear your seatbelt.
- Eat an apple on the drive home from work tonight.

As inspirational speaker Peter Lowe says, "You have the power to take the responsibility to change habits—limiting beliefs, self-defeating thoughts, and all the old excuses you used to justify your situation. You have the power to act in a different way. You do not have to be controlled by your own limiting beliefs and self-destructing thoughts on who you are or who you can be or what you can look like. Visualize and become a new and improved you."

Your quality of life begins today, with you and your lifestyle choices. You can redefine success and beauty as you travel through time. You are in control, and you can determine your future. The best is truly yet to come. You can feel fit and fabulous at any age. Right now you possess—in your own mind and body—everything you will ever need to be successful. You only have to believe in yourself to achieve your goals and dreams. Goals are only dreams put into a time frame, and the time frame for you is now! Just as you are, right where you are, you can succeed. Today, the choice is yours. Choose to be healthy, starting now. It is not too late to change your future. It is not too late to undo the past speckled with not-so-healthy choices. All that matters is today, this moment, and what choices you make in the future. What are you waiting for? You can look, feel, and be better in the future. Just give yourself a chance to succeed. Believe in yourself in order to achieve. You can do it.

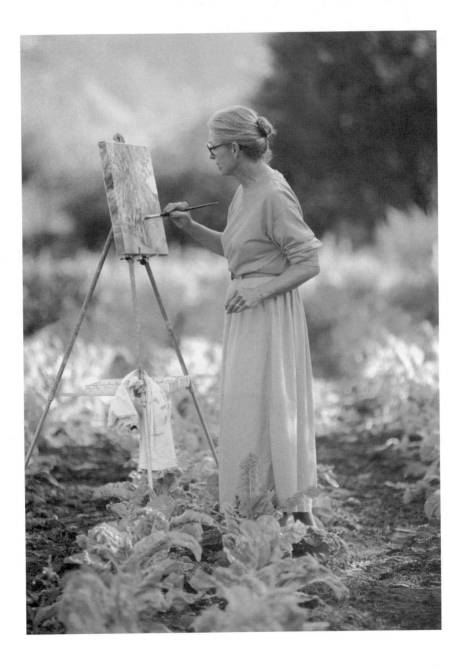

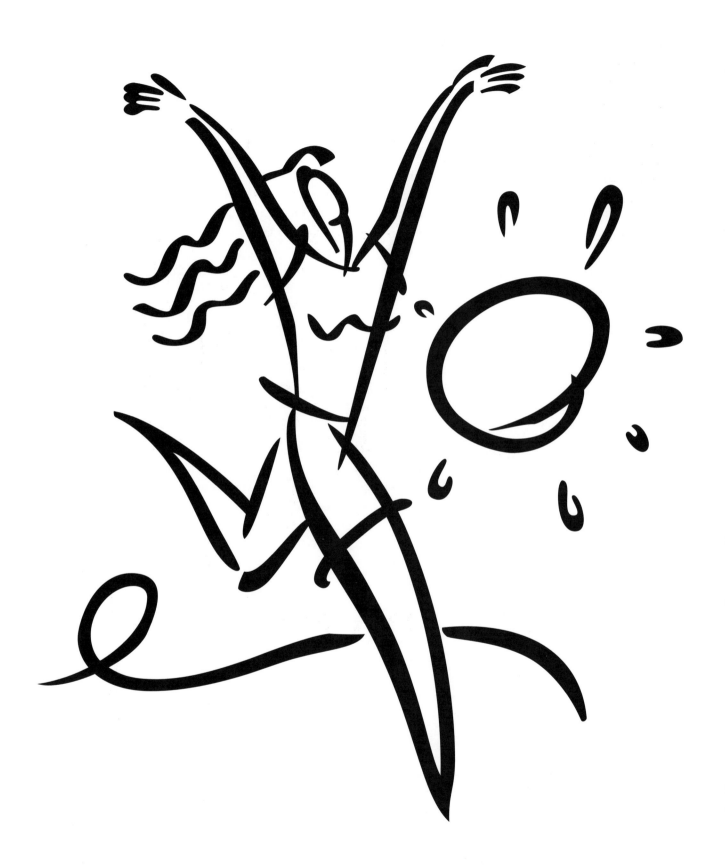

Glossary

A–C
Adeno: gland
ASC-US: a typical squamous cells of undetermined significance
Atrophy: shrunken cells
Baseline: measurement or calculation used as a basis for comparison
Colposcopy: microscope for the genital or cervix area
Contraindicated: medically inadvised
Curettage: scraping to get cells

D–G
Distal: anatomically located far from a point of reference (such as a point of attachment)
Dysplasia: abnormal cell change
Efficacy: effectiveness
Endo: inside
Epithelial: top (surface) cells
Extra: outside
Genetic expression: the way in which an individual's dominant and recessive genes manifest (hereditary illnesses, traits etc.)
Glandular: inside cells of uterus

H–L
HSIL: high-grade squamous intraepithelial lesion
In-situ: on surface
Intake Uterus: healthy, normal uterus
Intra Epithelial: inside surface cells
IU: international unit of measurement, based on accepted international standards
LSIL: low-grade intraepithelial lesion

M–R
mcg: microgram
Menses: menstruation (period)
mg: milligram
Morbidity: the relative incidence of disease
Reactive: cells showing a reaction
Reparative: repairing cells

S–U
Squamous: top tougher cells of vagina or cervix
Stat: immediately (often used in medical field)
Uteri: plural of uterus

References

Internet Resources

Aging
www.nih.gov/nia
Breast Health
www.bcra.nci.hih.gov/brc/
Diabetes
www.diabetes.org
Disease
www.cdc.gov
Health
www.healthfinder.org

www.aafp.org
Herbs
http://ods.od.nih.gov/databases/ibids.html

http://vm.cfsan.fda.gov/~dms/aems.html

http://dietary-supplements.info.nih.gov/

www.health.harvard.edu/newsletters

www.herbs.org/indes.html

www.ncrhi.org/main.html

nccam.nih.gov
Hormone Replacement Therapy
www.whi.org

www.jama.com

www.SalivaTest.com
Menopause
www.fda.gov/opacom/lowlit/menopause.html

www.menopause.org
Nutrition
www.fns.usda.gov/fns
Osteoporosis
www.nof.org
Pap Smears
www.bethesda2001.cancer/gov/terminology.html/
Perimenopause (and Menopause)
www.menopause.org

www.whi.org

http://bcra.nci.nih.gov/brc/

www.americanmenopause.org

www.nmh.org

www.cdc.gov/nccdphp/dnpa/bmi-for-age.htm

www.merkmedicus.com
Thyroid
www.thyroid.org
Urinary Incontinence
www.nafc.org
Vitamins
www.cc.nih.gov/ccc/supplements

www.navigator.tufts.edu
Weight Management
www.MayoClinic.com

www.shapeup.org

References

General

Phillips, Bill., and Michael D'Orso. *Body for Life*. New York: Harper Collins Publishers, 1999.

Thompson Medical Economics. *PDR Monthly Prescription Guide*. Montvale, New Jersey: N.p., 2002.

The Essential Women's Health Guide. Birmingham, Alabama: Time Inc. Health, 2000.

The Merck Manual, Seventh Edition. Whitehouse Station, New Jersey: Merck Research Laboratories, 1999.

Monthly Prescription Reference. N.p., 2001.

Wittels, Harriet and Joan Greisman. *The Clear and Simple Thesaurus Dictionary*. New York, New York: Scholastic Inc., 1996.

Diseases and Disorders. Skokie, Illinois: Anatomical Chart Company, 2000.

Cole, Raymond, D.O., CCD, CPT. *Best Body, Best Bones*. Brooklyn, Michigan: Wellpower Publications, 2001.

Breast/Ovary

"Scientific Basis for Accurate Detection of Ovarian Carcinoma, part 1." *The Female Patient* 27 (2002): 19–23.

Cauley, Jane, Dr., Ph.D. "Current and Future Directions in Breast Cancer Care." *The Female Patient*. (March 2002): 13–19.

United Health Care. *Breast Cancer Screening: Mammography*. N.p., 2002.

American Academy of Family Physicians. "Deciding About Mammography for Women Age 40–49." N.p., 2001.

Haberfelde, Mimi, R.N., M.S. "Breast Health." Stay Well featuring KRAMES. N.p., 1999.

"Screening for Breast Cancer: Recommendations and Rationale." *American Family Physicians* 65, no. 12 (2002): 2537–2543.

Keith, Louis G. and others. "Breast Cancer: An Equal Opportunity Killer." *The Female Patient* 26, no. 10 (2001): 15–26.

Eskin, Bernard A., M.S., M.D. and Vicken Sepilian, M.D. "Common Benign Conditions of the Breast." *The Female Patient* 26, no. 10 (October 2001): 35–40.

"New Issues in Breast Cancer." *Patent Care*. (May 2001): 40–60.

Fuqua, Suzanne, Ph.D. and others. "Selective Estrogen Receptor Modulators." N.p., 2001.

White, Melody, M.S. and others. "Breast and Ovarian Cancer Risk Assessment." N.p., 2002.

Colon Cancer

"Colorectal Cancer in Women." *JAOA* 12, no. 2 (December 2001 supplement): S8–S12.

Vick, Tara M., M.D. "Routine Screening for Cervical, Breast, and Colorectal Cancers." *The Female Patient* 27 (2002):20–24.

Depression

Archgen Psychiatry. *Zung Self-Rating Depression Scale*. N.p., 1999.

CME Express and Glaxo Wellcome Inc. *Primary Care Network*. N.p., 1999.

Glaxo Wellcome Inc. *Insights on Neurotransmitters*. N.p., 2000.

Prozac Weekly. *Depression: Staying on the Right Path*. Lilly, N.d.

Bristol-Meyers Squibb Company. *Track your Progress with BuSpar*. N.p., 1997.

Berges, Ronald, R., D.O. *PMDD and Depression - Optimum Treatment Strategies*.

Zung, William, M.D. *The Measurement of Depression*. Eli Lilly and Company, 1998.

Diet

Curtis, Brian M., M.D. and James H. O'Keefe, M.D., "Understanding the Meditterranean Diet." *Prostgraduate Medicine* 112, no. 2 (August 2002): 35–44.

Brownell, Kelly D., Ph.D. and Wadden, Thomas A., Ph.D. *The Learn Program for Weight Control*. American Health Publishing Company, 1999.

Pennington, Jean, A.T. *Food Values of Portions Commonly Used, Sixteenth Edition*. Philidelphia, Pennsylvania: Bowes and Church's, JB Lippincott Company, 1994.

Exercise

Smith, R.M. "Nutrition 101: Choosing a Healthy Heart." *For Your Health* 8, no. 1 (2002): 6–7.

Ryan, Nolan. *The Nolan Ryan Fitness Guide*. N.p., n.d.

Eating Right for a Healthier Diet. Warner-Lambert Export. LTD, 1996.

Dowling, Elizabeth A. "How Exercise Affects Lipid Profile in Women." *The Physician and Sports Medicine* 29, no. 4 (September 2001): 45–52.

Hoechst-Roussell Pharmaceuticals Inc. *Walking: Patient Information Card*.

"How Fit Are You?" *The Walking Magazine*. (July/August 1990): 63–65.

Roos, Robert J. "The Surgeon General's Report. " *The Physician and Sports Medicine* 25, no. 4 (1997): 122–131.

"Are You in Shape? Step on This Scale." *Fit or Fat* 85 (May/June 1996).

Zimmerman, Gretchen L., Psy.D. and others. "A 'Stages of Change' Approach to Helping Patients Change Behavior." *American Family Physician*, 61, no. 5 (2000): 1409–14

Taylor, Michael. "Celebrate Everyday Victories." *Arthritis Today*. (May/June 2001): 42–48.

Waring, Nancy. "Dr. Dean O'Rnish's Low-Tech Approach to CAD." *Hippocrates*. (January 2001): 31–37.

"Does Physical Activity Prevent Cancer?" *BMJ USA* 1, no. 13 (2001).

Fiber

"Getting Enough Fiber in Your Diet." *Patient Care*. (November 1993): 53–58.

Metamucil. *Fiber Content Chart*. University of Minnesota Press, N.d.

Heart

Krauss, Ronald M., M.D. "Diet and Cardioprotection: Sorting Fact From Fiction." *Menopause Management*. (January/February 2002): 6–10.

"Studies in Postmenopausal Women Have Demonstrated Beneficial Effects on SERMs on Several New Makers of CVD." *The Female Patient*. (March 2002): 23–26.

Clearfield, Michael B., D.O. "Do We Really Need Another Set of Cholesterol Guidelines?" *JAOA* 102, no. 5 (2002): S6–S11.

"Executive Summary of the Third Report of the National Cholesterol Education Program (NCEP) Expert Panel on Detection, Evaluation, and Treatment of High Blood Cholesterol in Adults." *JAMA* 285, no 19 (2001): 2486–2497.

Parke-Davis. *Eating Right to a Healthier Heart*. N.p., 1996.

National Cholesterol Education Program, Parke-Davis, and Pfizer. *Close to the Heart*. N.p, n.d.

Bach, Amanda J. "Your Heart is in Your Hands!" *The Female Patient*. (April 2002): 1–5.

"High Blood Cholesterol: Detection, Evaluation, and Treatment." *National Cholesterol Education Program*. *National Institutes of Health*. (May 2001): 1–26.

"Heart Disease." *Patient Care*. (May 2001): 61–73.

 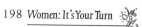

Garber, Alan J., M.D., Ph.D. "Attenuating Cardiovascular Risk Factors in Patients with Type 2 Diabetes." *American Family Physician* 62, no 12 (2000): 2633–2641.

"Cholesterol 2001, Rationale for Lipid-Lowering in Older Patients with or without CAD." *Geriatrics* 56, no 9 (2001): 22–25, 28–30.

"Primary Prevention of Ischemic Stroke." *AHA Scientific Statement* 103, no. 1 (2001): 163–177.

American Heart Association. *Controlling Your Risk Factors.*

Muchowski, Karen E., M.D. "Coronary Artery Disease in Women." *The Female Patient.* (June 2000): 27–31.

Iowa Heart Center. *Heart Disease: Are You at Risk?* N.p., n.d.

Wenger, Nanette K., M.D. "How to Keep Women's Hearts Healthy. Women's Health." *Primary Care* 5, no. 7 (2002): 432–441.

Wenger, Nanette K., M.D. "Preventing Coronary Heart Disease in Women: What You—and Your Patients—Can Do." *Consultant* 42, no.10 (2002): 1318–1324.

Pearlman, Brian L., M.D. F.A.C.P. "The New Cholesterol Guidelines." *Postgraduate Medicine* 112, no. 2 (2002): 13–26.

Herbs

PDR for Herbal Medicines. First Edition Montvale, New Jersey: Medical Economics Co., Inc, 1998.

Hormone Replacement Therapy (See also Natural Hormone Replacement Therapy)

Sagario, Dawn. "Frantic Women Storm Doctors with Questions." *The Des Moines Register,* 18 July 2002, Iowa Life Section.

Pfizer Inc. *Know the Facts on Menopause, Breast Cancer, and HRT.* N.p., 2001.

Pfizer Inc. *How Menopause Effects You.* N.p., 2001.

Pfizer Inc. *Learn About Menopause and HRT.* N.p., 2001.

Speroff, Lean, M.D. "Hormone Replacement and Breast Cancer." *The Female Patient.* (December 2001): 6–11.

French, Linda, M.D. "Approach to the Perimenopausal Patient." *The Journal of Family Practice* 51, no. 3 (March 2002): 271–276.

Shulman, Lee P., M.D. "Transdermal HRT: New Trends, Emerging Targets." *Contemporary OB/GYN,* (March 2002).

"Hormone Replacement Therapy. Relieving Symptoms of Menopause." San Bruno, California: The Stay Well Company, 2000.

Phillips, Owen P., M.D. "Raloxifene Versus Standard Hormone Replacement." *The Female Patient* 27 (May 2002): 32–36.

Barton, Debra L., R.N., Ph.D. and others. "Managing Hot Flashes: Findings on Alternatives to Traditional Hormone Therapy." *Menopause Management* 11, no. 3 (2002): 15–19.

"Managing Menopause: New Practice Guidelines." *Women Health Primary Care* 3, no. 8 (N.d.).

Krantz, Colleen. "Risks Seen in Hormone Therapy." *The Des Moines Register,* 10 July, 2002, Section A.

"A Quick-Reference Guide to Hormone Replacement Therapies." *International Journal of Pharmaceutical Compounding* 5, no. 5 (2001): 333–335.

Yanni, Leanne, M.D. and Wendy Klein, M.D. "Alternatives to Traditional Hormone Replacement Therapy." *Women's Health* 3, no. 7 (2000): 477–485.

Lacey, James Jr., Ph.D. "Menopausal HRT and Risk of Ovarian Cancer." *JAMA* 288, no. 3 (2000): 334–341.

Dull, Pamela, M.D. and others. "Phytoestrogens: A Women's Alternative to Estrogen Therapy." *Family Practice Recertification* 22, no. 15 (2000): 58–67.

Dysert, Gary, M.D. "Women interested in Risks and Benefits of HRT." *Family Practice Recertification* 22, no. 11 (2002): 13.

Gelfand, Morrie M., CM, M.D. "Estrogen-Androgen Therapy." *The Female Patient* 26 (September 2001): 45–46.

Kaunitz, Andrew M., M.D. "Reduced-Dose Oral Contraceptives." *The Female Patient* 26 (September 2001): 24–31.

"Hormone Replacement Therapy and the Breast." *BMJ USA* 2 (February 2002): 70–72.

Messinger-Rapport, Barbara, M.D., Ph.D. and Holly L. Thacker, MD. "Preventions for the Older Woman." *Geriatrics* 56, no. 9 (September 2001): 32–42.

Writing Group for Women's Health Organization. "Risks and Benefits of Estrogen Plus Progestin in Healthy Postmenopausal Women." *JAMA* 288, no. 3 (2002): 321–333.

"Oral Estrogens." *Patient Care.* (May 2001): 101–102.

"Answers to Some of Your Questions About Hormone Replacement Therapy." Wyeth-Ayerst Lab. March 1998.

Simon, James A., M.D. and Carol J. Mack, M.P.H. "Preventing Osteoporosis and Improving Compliance with HRT." *Patient Care.* (October 2001): 3–9.

Herrington, David M., M.D. "Understanding the Latest Data on HRT and Cardiovascular Health." *Patient Care.* (October 2001): 10–17.

Legro, Richard, M.D. and others. Women and Menopause Educational Initiative. *Individualized Hormone Therapy to Promote Better Health and Quality of Life.* N.p., 1999.

Johnson, Cynda, M.D. and David Archer, M.D. *Hormone Replacement Therapy: The Benefits and the Concerns.* The American of Family Physicians, 2000.

"Controversial Issues in Climacteric Medicine II: Hormone Replacement Therapy and Cancer." *Menopause Management* 10, no. 6 (2001): 8–20.

Speroff, Leon. "The Case for Postmenopausal Hormone Therapy. What Women Should Know About: The Body of Evidence Concerning Menopause and its Associated Estrogen Loss." *Hospital Practice* (1996).

Battistini, Michelle, M.D. and Heidi Stanley, Ph.D. "Complete Care of the Older Woman." *Patient Care.* (May 2001): 23–26.

Archer, David, M.D. and Wulf Utian, M.D. "Decisions in Prescribing HRT." *Patient Care.* (May 2001): 91–105.

Speroff, Lean and Ernest L. Mazzaferri. "Hormone Replacement Therapy: Clarifying the Picture." *Hospital Practice* (May 2001): 37–96.

Fiorica, James V., M.D. "The Impact of Hormone Replacement Therapy on Mammography." *Women's Health.* (October 2001): 13–16.

Blackwook, Michele, M.D. and others. "Postmenopausal Hormone Therapy: Informed Patients, Shared Decisions." *Women's Health.* (October 2001): 28–34.

Lockwood, Charles J., M.D. "Is Hormone Replacement Therapy Good for the Heart?" *Contemporary OB/GYN* 46 (September 2001): 4–5.

Apgar, Barbara S., M.D. *Managing the Perimenopause and Menopause.* N.p., n.d.

Johnson, Karen C., M.D. "Hormone Replacement and Cardiovascular Disease." *The Female Patient.* (October 2001): 5–8.

"Contemporary Issues in Hormone Replacement Therapy." *Mayo.* (January 2002).

Femhrt. Pfizer. *Help her Stay in Control of Menopause.* 2000.

Speroff, Leon, M.D. "The Impact of Low-Dose HRT." *Menopause Management.* (July 2001): 4–25.

Hormone Replacement Therapy: Multiple Benefits for Postmenopausal Women. Chicago, Illinois: Clinician's Group, LLC., A Jobson Company, 2001.

Collins, Geneva. "A Tailored Approach to Hormone Replacement Therapy." *The Female Patient.* (N.d.)

Speroff, Leon, M.D. "Postmenopausal HRT and CHD: Clinical Implications of Recent randomized Trial Results." *Contemporary OB/GYN.* (March 2001): 17–24.

"Raloxifene FAQ's: Perspectives on the First Approved SERM- Where Are We Now?" *Menopause Management.* (March/April 2001): 21–29.

Jaret, Peter. "What to Tell Patients About HRT." *Hippocrates.* (December 2000): 27–31.

Utian, Wulf H. "Hormone Replacement Therapy and Coronary Disease - Where Now?" *Menopause Management.* (November/December 2000): 7–8.

Simon, James A., M.D. "Unscheduled Bleeding During Continuous Combined HRT." *Menopause* 8, no. 5 (2001): 321–326.

Lorentzen, Jean. *Perspectives of Hormone Replacement Therapy.* N.p., n.d.

Lee, John R., M.D. *Saliva vs. Serum or Plasma Testing For Progesterone.* N.p., n.d.

Marshall, John R. M.D. "A Review of Current/Future Hormonal Contraceptives: A Focus on Progestins." *Medical Educaion Resources, Inc.* (September 2002): 1–10.

Yanni, Leanne, M.D. and Wendy Klein, MD. "Alternatives to Traditional Hormonal Replacement Therapy." *Women's Health in Primary Care* 7 (2000): 477–489.

"Managing Menopause: New Practice Guidelines." *Women's Health in Primary Care* 3, no. 8 (2000): 547–552.

Fletcher, Suzanne, M.D., MSC., "Failure of Estrogen Plus Progestin Therapy for Prevention." *JAMA* 288, no. 3 (2002): 366–7

Jeri, Auturo, M.D. "The Use of Isoflavone Supplement to Relieve Hot Flashes." *The Female Patient* 27 (2002): 47–49.

Pfizer Pharmaceuticals, Inc. *Hormone Replacement Therapy Prescribing Guide.* Montvale, New Jersey: Medical Economics Company, 2002.

Wright, Jonathan V., M.D. *Natural Hormone Replacement.* Petaluma, California: Smart Publications, 1997.

Hypo/Hyper Glycemia

Lilly. *Low Blood Sugar (hypoglycemia).* N.p, n.d.

Libido

Glaxo Wellcome. *Arizona Sexual Experiences Scale.* N.p., 1999.

Crossman, Jody. "Another (ahem) Toy Story." *The Des Moines Register,* 5 February, 2002, Iowa Life Section.

Shulman, Lee, M.D. "Female Sexual Dysfunction." *The Female Patient.* (December 2000): 3–8.

Freedman, Murray, M.D. and others. "Common Sexual Complaints." *The Female Patient.* (December 2000): 9–18.

Sarrel, Philip M., M.D. "Sexual Dysfunction and the Menopausal Woman: Overcoming Atrophic Vaginitis." *Patient Care.* (January 2002): 4–20.

"Female Sexual Dysfunction: Diagnosis and Treatment in 2002." *Patient Care.* (February 2002): 15–24.

Dell, Diana, M.D. "Female Sexual Dysfunction." *The Female Patient* 27, no. 3 (2002): 25–30.

Bachman, Gloria, M.D. Personal Evolution. *The Female Patient.* (December 2000): 5–11.

Renshaw, Domeena, M.D. "Theraputic Options." *The Female Patient Supplement.* (December 2000): 12–18

Kaplan, Steven, M.D. "Female Sexual Dysfunction: Diagnosis and Treatment in 2002." *Patient Care.* (February 2002): 15–24.

Make Over

Litt, Jerome Z., M.D. "Common Skin Problems in Older Women." *The Female Patient* 27 (2002): 35–38.

Walgreens. "Just Beach-y, A Summer Care Guide: Look Good Feel Good." N.p., (2002).

Menopause

Rymer, Janice and Edward P. Morris. "Menopausal Symptoms." *Clinical Review* 1 (2000): 60–64.

Van Amerongen, Derek, M.D., M.S. "Menopause in Managed Care." *Women's Health in Primary Care* 3, no. 12 (2000): 3

Cochran, Neva, M.S., R.D. "Eating Your Way Through Menopause." *The Female Patient.* 23–24.

Fugate, Woods, Nancy, R.N., Ph.D., F.A.A.N. and Ellen Mitchell Sullivan, Ph.D, A.R.N.P. "Menopause Transition." *The Female Patient* 25 (2001): 45–46.

Sagario, Dawn. "Is it Menopause?" *The Des Moines Register,* 10 December, 2001, Iowa Life Section.

Holstein, Lana L., M.D. "Enhancing the Sexual Connection in Midlife Women: The Clinician's Role." *Menopause Management* 10, no. 5 (2001): 15–23.

Mort, Elizabeth A., M.D., M.P.H. "HEDIS and Menopause Counseling: The Management of Menopause Measure." *Menopause Management* 10 no. 5 (2001): 8–12.

"News Briefs." *Menopause Management* 10, no. 5 (2001) 28–32.

Wyeth-Ayerst Laboratories. *Taking Charge of Your Menopause. Your Patient Action Guide.* N.p, 2001.

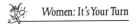

Cutson, Tomi M., M.D., M.H.S. and Emily Meuleman, M.S., R.N.C. "Managing Menopause." *American Family Physician* 61, no. 5 (2000): 1391–1400.

"Learning About Menopause: Information from your Family Doctor." *American Academy of Family Physicians* 61, no. 5 (2000): 1–2.

Speroff, Leon, M.D. "Management of the Perimenopausal Transition." *Contemporary OB/GYN*. (September 2000): 11–22.

Utian, Wulf H. "Managing Menopause After HERS II and WHI: Coping with the Aftermath." *Menopause Management*. (July/August 2002): 6–7.

Menses

Speroff, Lean, M.D. "Management of the Perimenopausal Transition." *Contemporary OB/GYN*. (September 2000): 11–23.

Natural Hormone Replacement Therapy

Lorentzen, Jean, D.O. *Perspective of Hormone Replacement Therapy*. N.p., n.d.

Wright, Jonathan, M.D. and John Morgenthaler. "Natural Hormone Replacement for women over 45." Petaluma, California: Smart Publications, 1997.

Hudson, Tori, N.D. "Natural Progesterone." *The Family Patient* 26 (April 2001): 32, 37–41.

Revis, Elaine S., Ph.D. and Claude L. Hughes, M.D. Ph.D. "Phytoestrogens and Women's Health: How Should We Advise Our Patients?" *Menopause Management*. (November/December 2000): 12–21.

Saunders, Carol S. "Sorting out health claims about soy." *Patient Care*. (December 2000): 14–28.

Hudson, Tori, N.D. "Soy and Women's Health." *The Female Patient* 26 (2001): 24–27.

Zava, David, P.h.D. *Hormonal Balance and Your Health*. Beaverton, Oregon: N.p., n.d.

Zava, David, P.h.D. *Steroid Hormone Overview*. Beaverton, Oregon: N.p., 1999.

"Saliva Vs. Serum or Plasma Testing for Progesterone." *The John R. Lee, M.D. Medical Letter: Special Report*.

Zava, David, P.h.D. "About Hormones." N.p., 1999.

Horton, Sue, R.Ph. and Carolyn Walker, M.S.N, A.R.P. *Natural Hormone Replacement Therapy*. N.p., n.d.

Ahlgrimm, Marla, R.Ph. *Natural Hormone Replacement Therapy*. Madison, Wisconsin: N.p., 2000.

Nutrition

James F. Balch, M.D. and Phyllis A. Balch, C.N.C. *Prescription for Nutritional Healing*. Garden City Park, New York: Avery Publishing Group, 1997.

Bauer, Joy. "The 10% Solution." *Readers Digest*. (January 2002): 97–103.

Dietary Guidelines for Americans: Aim for Fitness, Build a Healthy Base. *Home and Garden Bulletin*, no. 232 (2002): 2–39.

Nutrition Strategies: Designs for Heart-Healthy Living. Chicago, Illinois: Natural Livestock and Meat Board, 1995.

Healthy Choices: Diet for a Healthy Heart. Chicago, Illinois: Natural Livestock and Meat Board, 1989.

"Eating Smart When Your Pressed for Time." Chicago, Illinois: Education Department of National Cattlemen's Beef Association, 1996.

"Diet, Nutrition, and Cancer Prevention: A Guide to Food Choices." *US Department of Health and Human Services*. (May 1987): 1–39.

US Department of Agriculture. *Food Guide Pyramid: A Guide to Daily Food Choices*. N.p., 1993.

Food in Focus: A Nurse's Guide to Nutrition. N.p., 1991.
Bray, George A., M.D. "Obesity: Is There Effective Treatment?" *Consultant*. (July 2002): 1014–1020.

Jaret, Peter. "Are Nurtaceuticals Any Good?" *Hippocrates*. (March 1998): 62–67.

Beecham Laboratories. "Planning Means to Lose Weight: Guidelines for Systematic Slimming." N.p., n.d.

 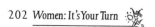

"Cholesterol Testing and Management: Updated Guidelines." *Consultant.* (September 2001): 1399–1403.

Carper, Jean. "6 Secret Disease-Fighters." *USA Weekend,* 2 January-February, 1997.

Monk, Arlene, R.D., C.D.E. "How to Avoid Yo-Yo Diet Syndrome." *Diabetes in the News.* (February 1991): 22–23.

"Getting Enough Fiber in Your Diet." *Patient Care.* (November 1993): 53–56.

Osteoporosis

Dore, Robin, K. "Osteoporosis: Fractures and Key Risk Factory." *The Female Patient Supplement.* (March 2002): 5-12.

Hodgson, Stephen, and others. *AACE 2001 Guidelines for Prevention and Management of Postmenopausal Osteoporosis.* Madison, Wisconsin: Health America Group.

Endocrine Practice, no.4 (July/August 2001): 293–312.

Lindsay, Robert and others. "Effect of Lower Doses of Conjugated Equine Estrogens with and without Medroxyprogesterone Acetate on Bone in Early Postmenopausal Women." *JAMA* 287, no. 20 (2002): 2668–2676.

Khan, MZ, M.D. and others. "Osteoporosis: What to Tell Patients About Prevention and Treatment." *Consultant.* (April 2002): 597–601.

Barrett, Conner E. and others. "Raloxifene and Cardiovascular Events in Osteoporotic Postmenopausal Women." *JAMA* 287, no. 7 (2002): 847–857.

Duvall, K. "Advances in the Prevention and Management of Osteoporosis." *FPR* 23, no. 13 (2001): 19–24.

United Health Care. *Osteoporosis Screening.* N.p., 2002.

"Mercy Arthritis and Osteoporosis" Des Moines, Iowa: Mercy Medical Center, n.d.

"Referring Women to Bone Densitometry." *Women's Health in Primary Care* 5, no. 1 (2002): 37–38.

Liberman, Uri A., M.D., Ph.D. "Effect of Oral Alendronate on Bone Mineral Density and the Incidence of Fractures in Postmenopausal Osteoporosis." *The New England Journal of Medicine.* (1995): 1437–1443.

Cummings, Steven R., M.D. "Effect of Alendronate on Risk of Fracture in Women With Low Bone Density but Without Vertebral Fractures." *JAMA* 280, no. 24 (1998): 2077–2081.

Yonclas, Peter, M.D. and Todd P., M.D. "How Much Exercise is Enough for Bone Health?" *Consultant* 42, no. 7 (2002) 829–833.

"Taking Charge of Your Menopause: Straight Facts About Menopause, Estrogen Loss, and Your Body. " N.d., August 2001.

Lilly. The Evista Woman: At Risk for Osteoporosis. N.p., 2002.

The Threat of Osteoporosis:What you can do about the threat of bone loss, osteoporosis, and resulting fracture in postmenopausal women. N.p., 2001.

Faulkner, Kenneth G., Ph.D. and Sydney L. Bonnick, M.D. "Clinical Use of Bone Densitometry." *The American Journal of Medicine.* (2001): 1–10.

"The Medical Letter on Drugs and Therapeutics." Volume 42. (2000): 97–100.

"Effects of Risedronate Treatment on Vertebral and Nonvertebral Fractures in Women With Postmenopausal Osteoporosis." *JAMA* 282, no. 14 (1999): 1344–1352.

Siris, Ethel S., M.D. "Identification and Fracture Outcomes of Undiagnosed Low Bone Mineral Density in Postmenopausal Women." *JAMA* 286, no. 22 (2001): 2815–2822.

Chestnut III, Charles H., M.D. "Osteoporosis, an Under Diagnosed Disease." *JAMA* 286, no. 22 (2001): 2865–2866.

Lindsay, Robert. and Pierre J. Meunier. *Osteoporosis International* 11, no. 1 (2000): 83–91.

McClung, Michael R., M.D. and Piet Geusens, M.D. "Effect of Risedronate on the Risk of Hip Fracture in Elderly Women." *The New England Journal of Medicine* 334, no. 5 (2001).

Lanza, Frank L. and others. "Endoscopic Comparison of Esophageal and Gastroduodenal Effects of Risedronate and Alendronate in Postmenopausal Women." *Alimentary Tract* 119 (2000): 631–638.

" Therapeutic Equivalence of Alendronate 70 mg Once Weekly and Alendronate 10 mg Daily in the Treatment of Osteoporosis." *Aging Clinician* 12, no. 1 (2000): 1–12.

American Association of Clinical Endocrinologists. *Stand Strong against Osteoporosis.* N.p., 2001.

Rooney, Theodore, D.O. *Osteoporosis.* N.p., n.d.

Chestnut III, Charles, M.D. "The Concept of Bone Quality." *Osteoporosis Management Today* 1, no. 2 (1999): 1–4.

"The Bone Quality Concept: Implications to Fracture Risk in Osteoporosis." Sitges, Spain International experts meeting, March 5-7, 1999.

"Osteoporosis A Clinical Perspective." *The West Central Osteoporosis Board*, no. 4 (August 2001).

Cadarette, Suzanne M., M.S.C and others. "Evaluation and Decision Rules for Referring Women for Bone Density by Dual-Energy X-Ray Absorptiometry." *JAMA* 286, no. 1 (2001): 57–63.

Silverman, Lindsay R. and others. "Risk of New Vertebral Fracture in the Year Following a Fracture." *JAMA.* (January 2001).

South-Paul, Jeannette. "Nonpharmacologic and Pharmacologic Treatment." *American Family Physician* 63, no. 6 (2001): 1121–1128.

South-Paul, Jeannette. "Evaluation and Assessment." *American Family Physician* 63, no. 5 (2001): 897–904.

Pfizer. Femhrt. *Help Your Menopausal Patients Stay Strong: the Facts on Osteoporosis, Menopause, and HRT.* N.p., 2001.

Miller, Paul D., M.D. "Current Controverseries in Bone Densitometry." *Menopause Management.* (May/June 2001): 20–26.

"Preventing Bone Loss." *Patient Care.* (May 2001): 75–86.

"Women's Health News." *Contemporary OB/GYN.* (March 2001): 35–38.

"Clinical Inquiries." *The Journal of Family Practice* 59, no. 12 (2001): 1023–1025.

Proctor and Gamble Pharmaceuticals. *Actonal for the Prevention and Treatment of Postmenopausal and Glucocorticoid-Induced Osteoporosis.* N.p., n.d.

National Osteoporosis Foundation. *Physician's Guide to Prevention and Treatment of Osteoporosis: Update on Medications.* N.p., 2002.

Cole, Raymond E., D.O., CCD. *Osteoporosis: Unmasking a Silent Thief.* Brooklyn, Michigan: Wellpower Publications, 2000.

Cole, Raymond E., D.O., CCD. *Osteoporosis: Unmasking a Silent Thief.* Brooklyn, Michigan: Wellpower Publications, 2000.

Pap Smears

United Healthcare Inc. *Cervical Cancer Screening. Clinical Practice Measure Overview.* N.p., 2001.

Krames Health and Safety Education. Abnormal Pap Test Results: Understanding Your Diagnosis and Management Options. San Bruno, California: Stay Well Publications, 2000, 2001.

"Pap Testing: Advances in Cervical Cancer Screening." *Contemporary OB/GYN.* (September 2001): 3–18.

Videldsky, A., M.D. and others. "Routine Vaginal Cuff Smear Testing In Post Hysterectomy Patient with Benign Uterine Conditions: When is it Indicated?" *JABFP* 13, no. 4 (2000): 233–238.

The Bethesda Conference. September 6–9, 2001.

NCI *Bethesda System.* N.p., 2001.

Bethesda System for Reporting Cervical/Vaginal Cytological Diagnoses. N.p., 1988.

Premenstrual Syndrome References

Sarafem for PMDD. *Premenstrual Daily Symptom Chart.* N.p., n.d.

Hudson, Tori, N.D. "Premenstrual Syndrome, Part 1." *The Female Patient* 27 (2002): 37–39.

Yuzpe, Albert, M.D., M.S.C, F.R.C.S. "Contraception and Quality of Life: PMS/PMDD and Other Patient Concerns." *Beyond Contraception: Enhancing the Quality of Life.* (March 2002): 9–12.

 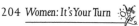

Prevention

"Summary of Policy Recommendations for Periodic Health Examinations." Rev. 5.1, *American Academy of Family Physicians.* (December 2001): 2–15.

Zoorob, Roger, M.D., M.P.H and others. "Cancer Screening Guidelines." *American Family Physician* 63, no. 6 (2001): 1101–1112.

Bial, Andrea K., M.D. and Daniel Brauner, M.D. "Cancer Screening in the Elderly: Which, When and Why." *Family Practice Recertification* 24, no. 8 (2001) 18–37.

Friedman, Jodi, M.D. "Cancer Screening in Premenopausal Women." *Family Practice Recertification* 24, no. 1 (2002): 53–62.

"Colorectal and Endometrial Cancers: ACS Guidelines for Early Detection." *Women's Health* 4, no. 6 (2001): 421–424.

Wolf, Andrew, M.D. "Cancer Prevention and Early Detection." *Consultant.* (May 2001): 911–917.

Gates, Thomas J., M.D. "Screening for Cancer: Evaluating the Evidence." *American Family Physician* 63, no. 3 (2001): 513–522.

Mayfield, Eleanor. "Celebrate a Year of Good Health at Any Age." *The Female Patient.* (September 2000): 4–12.

Wellmark Health Plan of Iowa. Your Arch and Sole: Take Care of Your Feet. *Well-being.* (Fall 2001): 12–14.

Pfizer Inc. *The Women's Health Datebook: Information for Women Ages 21–50.* N.p., 1999.

Medicare Preventive Service Benefits. December 1997.

National Institutes of Health, National Heart, Lung, and Blood Institute. *The JNCVI Guide to Prevention and Treatment of Hypertension Recommendations.* N.p., 1997.

Redefine Success

American Heart Association. *Fitting Fitness In Even When Your Pressed for Time.* N.p., 1996.

Adipex-P. *Patient Support Program Exercise.* N.p., 1992.

Adipex-P. *Exercise Calories Expended.* N.p., n.d.

Frank, Arthur, M.D. "Diet and Exercise: Guidelines for Weight Management." *Family Practice Recertification* 22, no. 5 (2000): 7–12.

Wadden, Thomas A., Ph.D. "Patient Counseling on Weight Management." *Family Practice Recertification* 22, no. 5 (April 2000): 22–26.

Heber, David, M.D., Ph.D. "Fat Metabolism Throughout the Life Cycle." *The Female Patient* 26 (April 2001): 16–25.

Sex

Nachtigall, Lila, M.D. "Sexuality in Menopause: Sexual Disfunction and Menopause." *Women's Health in Primary Care.* (August 2002): 4–14.

Spirit, Mind, and Body

Bortz, Walter, M.D. "Use It or Lose It." *Runners World.* (August 1990): 55–58.

Warner-Lambert Export, Ltd. "Eating Right For a Healthier Heart." N.p., 1996.

Colino, Stacey. "Lose Fat Faster." *McCall's.* (September 1995): 48–50.

American Academy of Family Physicians. *Weight Control: Losing Weight and Keeping it Off.* N.p., 1994.

Peter Lowe's TWA Success Seminar. Peter Lowe International. 1999. Convention Center, Des Moines, Iowa.

Skin Cancer

Nagelberg, Jilleyn. "Melanoma, a Year-Round Danger." *The Family Patient.* (April 2002): 12–13.

Let the Sun Shine: Take Steps to Prevent Skin Cancer. Yardley, Pennsylvania: Triple, 2002.

Walgreens. *Just Beach-y, A Summer Care Guide,* 2002.

Style References

"Great Picks." *USA Weekend*. March 2002.

Totten, Priscilla. "Why Fashion Matters." *USA Weekend*. 29–31 March, 2002.

Thyroid References

Siperstein, Allan, M.D. *Medical and Surgical Treatment of Thyroid Problems: The Thyroid Book*. San Bruno, California: The Stay Well Corp., 2001.

Bour, Alison M. "Thyroid Disease and Genetics, Knowing the Risk." *The Female Patient*. (June 2002): 1–4.

Cohen, Harvey D., M.D. and Karen L. Levanduski-Cohen, M.S. "Thyroid Disorders." *The Female Patient* 27. (2002): 30–34.

Collins, Geneva. "Thyroid Disease: When Your Body's Regulator Goes Awry." *The Female Patient*. 21–24.

Grardner, David F., M.D. "Thyroid Disease: When the Screen: How to Avoid Treatment Pitfalls." *Ask the Professor*. (December 2000): 2397–2401.

Laboratory of Clinical Medicine. Laboratory Test Guide to Thyroid Evaluation. Des Moines, Iowa: N.p., n.d.

Macindoe, John H., M.D. "Office Thyroidology: An Interactive Approach." University of Iowa College of Medicine: N.p., n.d.

Urine Incontinence References

Vardy, Michael, M.D. "Urinary Incontinence." *The Female Patient*. (June 2002): 7–16.

"Gimme a Pee!" *Sports Illustrated* 96, no. 10 (2002): 28.

Schiff, Isaac, M.D. "Your Patient and HRT: Strategies for Continuance in the Early Years." *Patient Care*. (May 2002): 4–19.

Davila, Willa G., M.D. and others. "Emerging Trends in the Management of Overactive Bladder." *Geriatrics* 57 (2002): 5–34.

"Menopause and Urinary Problems. The North American Menopause Society." *The Female Patient*. (June 2002): 11–12.

Rovner, Eric S. M.D. and Alan J. Wein. "The Treatment of Overactive Bladder in the Geriatric Patient." *Clinical Geriatrics* 10, no. 1 (January 2002): 20–32.

Wein, AJ., and ES Rovner. *Institute Journal of Infertility* 44, no. 2 (1999): 56–66.

Detrol LA. and Pharmacia Company. *Recent Advances in the Management of Overactive Bladder*. N.p., 2001.

Tunick, Barbara. "Hormones and Health: Living in Balance." *The Female Patient*. 4–7.

Ouslander, Joseph G. M.D. and others. "Overactive Bladder: New Treatment Options." *Clinical Geriatrics*. (November 2001 supplement). 1–13.

Dmochowski, Roger, M.D. "Recognition and Treatment of Overactive Bladder." *Family Practice Recertification* 23, no. 9 (July 2001): 19–30

Culligan, Patrick, M.D. and Michael Heit, M.D. "Urinary Incontinence in Women: Evaluation and Management." *American Family Physician* 62, no. 11 (December 2000): 2433–2443.

Incontinence and Overactive Bladder: A Common and Treatable Condition. San Bruno, California: Stay Well Company, n.d.

Vaginal/ Vulvar References

Sarrel, Philip M., M.D. "Sexual Dysfunction and the Menopausal Woman: Case Studies in Atrophic Vaginitis." *Patient Care*. (April 2002): 4–9.

Sarrel, Philip, M.D. "Overcoming Atrophic Vaginitis." *Patient Care*. (January 2002): 4–19.

Galask, R. M.D. and Mary Fraser, R.N. *Guidelines for Vulvar Skincare*. N.p., 1991.

Vitamins

Fairfield, Kathleen and Robert Fletcher, M.D. "Vitamins for Chronic Disease Prevention in Adults." *JAMA* 287, no. 23 (2002): 3116–3129.

Prevention. *Guide to Vitamins and Minerals*. Emmaus, Pennsylvania: Rodale Press Inc., 1987.

Everette, Lisa, R.ph., F.A.C.A. *A Therapeutic Approach to Nutrition.* N.p., 2000.

"Herbal Remedies." *Emergency Medicine.* (May 2002): 37–39.

Pennington, Jean, A.T. *Food Values of Portions Commonly Used.* 16th Ed. Philadelphia, Pennsylvania: Bowers and Churches. J.B. Lippincott Company, 1994.

Bauer, Brent, M.D. *Herbal Therapy.* N.p., 2001.

Davis, Lisa. "Custom-Fit Vitamins." *Reader's Digest.* (November 2001): 89–95.

Balch, James F. and Phyllis A. Balch. *Prescription for Nutritional Healing.* 2nd Ed. Garden City Park, New York: Avery Publishing Group, 1997.

Health Maintenance Chart

Date __/__/___

Name _____

Date of Birth __/__/___

Status: Married ☐   Single ☐   Divorced ☐   Widowed ☐

SBE Prophylaxis: Yes ☐   No ☐

Allergies

PM HX:

P SURG/HOSPITALIZATION

FAMILY HX _____

Mother _____

Father _____

MGM _____ PGM _____

MGF _____ PGF _____

Siblings _____

_____

_____

Children _____

_____

SOC HX: G__ P__ Contraception _____

Occupation _____

TOB _____

Coffee: Cups/day ___ Other caffeine _____

Alcohol _____ Drinks/day _____

Diet _____

Exercise _____

Seat belt use: Yes ☐ No ☐

Immunizations: ☐ See Immunization Form _____

Discussed: OTC Drug ☐   Sex Behavior ☐   Guns ☐

Helmets ☐   Sunscreen ☐   Water Heater Temp ☐

Smoke Alarm ☐

CO Alarm ☐ _____

CHRONIC MEDS:

EXAM:

Date/Results								
BP								
Weight								
Height								
Pap Smear								
Cholesterol								
TSH								
Colonoscopy								
Stool OB								
Flex Sig/BE								
CXR								
Mammogram								
Calcium Supp.								
Diet/Exer/Fiber								
Self Breast Exam								
Bone Density								

Advanced Directives: Yes ☐   No ☐   Date Discussed __/__/___   Received ☐   Living Will ☐

Durable Power of Attorney for Health Care   Organ Donor   Yes ☐   No ☐

On the following page is your **Health Maintenance Chart**. Below is an explanation of terms used on the chart, and how to fill out each section of the chart. This form is the same (or very similar) to the type of form your doctor fills out about you. Taking charge of your physical health includes taking charge of your medical history; make sure you are informed about your past and present medical condition. We have all gone to our doctor's office and wondered what they are writing on those charts—now you will know, and will be able to go to the doctor with your information ready.

Health Maintenance Chart Instructions

Section 1:
Fill in today's date, as well as your name, date of birth, and marital status. **SBE Prophylaxis** refers to whether or not you need an antibiotic before dental work (your doctor can fill in this part).

Section 2:
The Allergies section is where you list all of your allergies, including any allergies to medications or environment. (Ex. Penicillin or ragweed).

Section 3:
PM HX stands for past medical history. In this section you can include any significant medical health history. This could include such items as: pneumonia, mononucleosis, high blood pressure, fractures, diabetes, etc.

Section 4:
P SURG/HOSPITALIZATION is the section where you list any surgical procedures (in- or outpatient), and any hospitalizations you have had.

Section 5:
FAMILY HX is the section for family medical history; include information on whether or not the family members listed are living, and what major medical conditions they have/had. **MGM** represents maternal grandmother, **PGM** represents paternal grandmother, **MGF** represents maternal grandfather, and **PGF** represents paternal grandfather. This section is very important for you because it shows what diseases may be in your genetic makeup. (Ex. If you have three blood relatives who have/have had diabetes, you may want to be checked routinely for diabetes.)

Section 6:
CHRONIC MEDS is where you list any medications or over-the-counter products you take on a regular basis. (Ex. Calcium, multivitamin, insulin, blood pressure medicine and dosage.)

Section 7:
SOC HX is the section where you record your social history. **G** represents the number of pregnancies you have had, **P** represents the number of children you have had. Also in this section, list the types of contraception you have used/are using, what your occupation is, if you are a smoker (**TOB**) and how much you smoke per day, how many cups of coffee (or other caffeine) you consume per day, how many alcoholic drinks you consume per day, whether or not you have a balanced diet, what type of/how much exercising you do, and whether or not you use your seatbelt. You should also record whether or not you have had a tetanus shot as an adult, and the other immunizations you have had/may need. If you are not sure of your immunization status, your doctor will refer to your immunization form for more information. You may also discuss with your doctor which over-the-counter (**OTC**) drugs you are taking, your sexual behavior (monogamous, abstinent, etc.), if you own/use guns, your helmet use (for bicycles or motorcycles), whether or not you wear sunscreen, if you are careful to regulate your water heater temperature, and if you have working smoke and carbon monoxide (**CO**) alarms.

Section 8:
EXAM is the section where you can record the date and results of your last blood pressure (**BP**) check, weight check, height measurement, pap smear, cholesterol check, thyroid stimulating hormone (**TSH**) check, stool occult blood test (**OB**), flex sigmoidoscopy (**Flex Sig**)/barium enema (**BE**), chest X-ray (**CXR**), mammogram, self breast exam, bone density test, and colonoscopy. In this section, you can also record if you are taking a calcium supplement, and if your diet, exercise, and fiber intake are at exceptable levels. In the blank lines you can add any other health-related topics you think you should be monitoring. This section is separated into eight columns—one column per year; so, you can use one chart to monitor your health for eight years.

Section 9:
Advanced Directives refers to what type of care you would like to have if you become unable to make a medical decision (Ex. If you are in a coma). In this section you can also record on what date the advanced directives were last discussed with/received by your doctor, if you have a living will, if someone has durable power of attorney for your health care, and if you are an organ donor.

Staying Your Best: Health Maintenance Guidelines*

	30–39 years	40–49 years	50+ years
Physical Exam	Every 3–5 years	Every 2–3 years	Every 1–2 years
Height	Every 3–5 years	Every 2–3 years	Every 1–2 years
Weight	Every 3–5 years	Every 2–3 years	Every 1–2 years
Eyes	Every 1–2 years	Every 1–2 years	Every 1–2 years
Teeth	Every 6 months	Every 6 months	Every 6 months
Hearing	Age 60 (screen)		
Skin (self exam)	Monthly	Monthly	Monthly
Skin (doctor exam)	Yearly	Yearly	Yearly
Bones		Early screen if history (HX) of hysterectomy, family HX of osteoporosis, adult HX of fracures or low calcium intake or absporption	At least one screening bone density if postmenopausal
Heart*			
Blood Pressure	Every 2–3 years	Every 1–2 years	Every year
Cholesterol	Every 5 years	Every 3–5 years	Once, then every 2–3 years
LDL	Every 5 years	Every 3–5 years	Once, then every 2–3 years
Triglycerides	Every 5 years	Every 3–5 years	Once, then every 2–3 years
HDL	Every 5 years	Every 3–5 years	Once, then every 2–3 years
Diabetes*			
Blood Sugars	Every 3–5 years	Every 3–5 years	Once, then every 3 years (sooner if needed)
Shots			
Tetanus/Diptheria	Every 10 years	Every 10 years	Every 10 years
Influenza	If needed	If needed	Yearly
Pneumonia	If needed	If needed	Once at age 65
Breast			
(self exam)	Monthly	Monthly	Monthly
(clinical exam)	Yearly	Yearly	Yearly
Mammogram	Screen if family history	Every 1–2 yrs	Every year
PAP: cervical**	Every 1–3 years if three in a row are normal	Every 1–3 years if three in a row are normal	Every 1–3 years if always normal
Pelvic (vulvar, vagina, uterus, ovaries)	Every 1–3 years	Every 1–3 years	Every 1–3 years
Thyroid/TSH*	If symptomatic	If symptomatic	Once, then if symptomatic
CBC/UA* (anemia, bladder, kidney screen)	If symptomatic	Once, then if symptomatic	Once, then every 3 years
Colon			
Digital Rectal Exam	If symptomatic	If symptomatic	Yearly
Guaiac/Hemocult	If symptomatic	If symptomatic	Yearly
Flex sig/Barium Enema (BE)	If symptomatic	If symptomatic	Every 3–5 years with BE every 5–10 years
Colonoscopy	If symptomatic, or if increased risk then screening colonoscopy	If symptomatic, or if increased risk then screening colonoscopy	Every 5–10 years. If increased risk or history of polyps, then more frequently (3–5 years)

**For all labs and tests: if any are abnormal, or you have a disease state involving above, labs may need to be checked more frequently.

**Yearly pap if on birth control pill. If hysterectomy for cancer, abnormal cells, or for reasons unknown, then per doctor's orders.

Healthzone Plan: 21 Days to Success

Here is your 21-day plan to healthier living. It is easy to follow. Place these in a convenient location. Each pyramid represents one day in the 21-day plan. Each pyramid has boxes that represent the healthy amounts of serving sizes you should have each day for each category.

As you eat a serving of food, do some exercise, or do a positive thought, deed, or action, put a check mark in the box to keep track of your healthy choices. **Your goal is to have most boxes marked off most days.** Each day is a fresh start for a new you. Follow this plan for six days and then take a day off; then, continue the plan the next day. Feel rejuvenated and energized in 21 days. **The secret to your success is to eat a serving size of each of the foods that you select and to keep your body moving!**

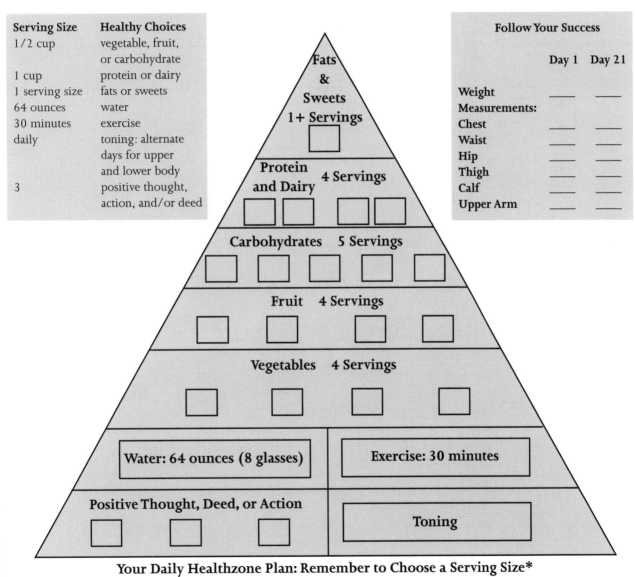

Your Daily Healthzone Plan: Remember to Choose a Serving Size*

*Pyramid based on a daily calorie intake consisting of 1400 calories a day. See "Daily Serving Sizes Suggested" chart on page 43 to create a Healthzone Plan based on a 1600 or 1800 daily calorie intake.

Food pyramid information adapted with permission from the "Mayo Clinic Healthy Weight Pyramid," © 2001 Mayo Foundation for Medical Education and Research, Rochester, Minnesota

DAY 1

Fats
&
Sweets

Protein
and Dairy

Carbohydrates

Fruit

Vegetables

Water: 64 ounces (8 glasses) | Exercise: 30 minutes

Positive Thought, Deed, or Action | Toning

DAY 2

Fats
&
Sweets

Protein
and Dairy

Carbohydrates

Fruit

Vegetables

Water: 64 ounces (8 glasses) | Exercise: 30 minutes

Positive Thought, Deed, or Action | Toning

DAY 3

Fats
&
Sweets

Protein
and Dairy

Carbohydrates

Fruit

Vegetables

Water: 64 ounces (8 glasses) | Exercise: 30 minutes

Positive Thought, Deed, or Action | Toning

DAY 4

Fats
&
Sweets

Protein
and Dairy

Carbohydrates

Fruit

Vegetables

Water: 64 ounces (8 glasses) | Exercise: 30 minutes

Positive Thought, Deed, or Action | Toning

DAY 5

Fats
&
Sweets

Protein
and Dairy

Carbohydrates

Fruit

Vegetables

Water: 64 ounces (8 glasses) | Exercise: 30 minutes

Positive Thought, Deed, or Action | Toning

DAY 6

Fats
&
Sweets

Protein
and Dairy

Carbohydrates

Fruit

Vegetables

Water: 64 ounces (8 glasses) | Exercise: 30 minutes

Positive Thought, Deed, or Action | Toning

**DAY 7 is a
FREE DAY**

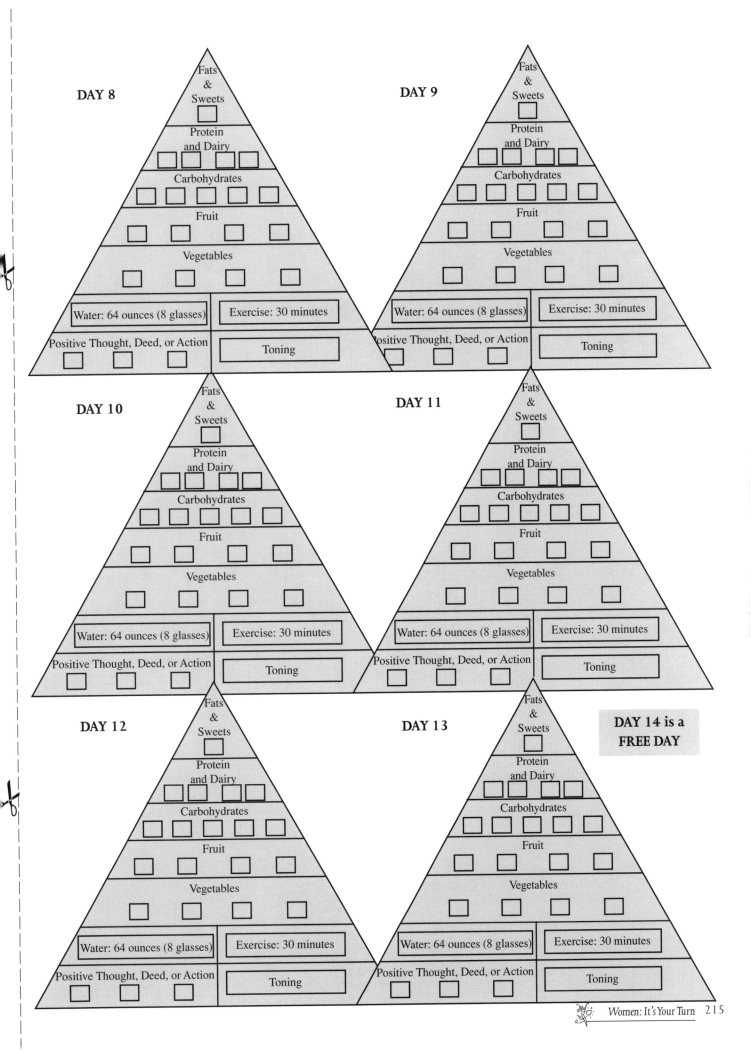

DAY 8

Fats & Sweets

Protein and Dairy

Carbohydrates

Fruit

Vegetables

Water: 64 ounces (8 glasses)

Exercise: 30 minutes

Positive Thought, Deed, or Action

Toning

DAY 9

Fats & Sweets

Protein and Dairy

Carbohydrates

Fruit

Vegetables

Water: 64 ounces (8 glasses)

Exercise: 30 minutes

Positive Thought, Deed, or Action

Toning

DAY 10

Fats & Sweets

Protein and Dairy

Carbohydrates

Fruit

Vegetables

Water: 64 ounces (8 glasses)

Exercise: 30 minutes

Positive Thought, Deed, or Action

Toning

DAY 11

Fats & Sweets

Protein and Dairy

Carbohydrates

Fruit

Vegetables

Water: 64 ounces (8 glasses)

Exercise: 30 minutes

Positive Thought, Deed, or Action

Toning

DAY 12

Fats & Sweets

Protein and Dairy

Carbohydrates

Fruit

Vegetables

Water: 64 ounces (8 glasses)

Exercise: 30 minutes

Positive Thought, Deed, or Action

Toning

DAY 13

Fats & Sweets

Protein and Dairy

Carbohydrates

Fruit

Vegetables

Water: 64 ounces (8 glasses)

Exercise: 30 minutes

Positive Thought, Deed, or Action

Toning

DAY 14 is a FREE DAY

DAY 15

Fats & Sweets

Protein and Dairy

Carbohydrates

Fruit

Vegetables

Water: 64 ounces (8 glasses) | Exercise: 30 minutes

Positive Thought, Deed, or Action | Toning

DAY 16

Fats & Sweets

Protein and Dairy

Carbohydrates

Fruit

Vegetables

Water: 64 ounces (8 glasses) | Exercise: 30 minutes

Positive Thought, Deed, or Action | Toning

DAY 17

Fats & Sweets

Protein and Dairy

Carbohydrates

Fruit

Vegetables

Water: 64 ounces (8 glasses) | Exercise: 30 minutes

Positive Thought, Deed, or Action | Toning

DAY 18

Fats & Sweets

Protein and Dairy

Carbohydrates

Fruit

Vegetables

Water: 64 ounces (8 glasses) | Exercise: 30 minutes

Positive Thought, Deed, or Action | Toning

DAY 19

Fats & Sweets

Protein and Dairy

Carbohydrates

Fruit

Vegetables

Water: 64 ounces (8 glasses) | Exercise: 30 minutes

Positive Thought, Deed, or Action | Toning

DAY 20

Fats & Sweets

Protein and Dairy

Carbohydrates

Fruit

Vegetables

Water: 64 ounces (8 glasses) | Exercise: 30 minutes

Positive Thought, Deed, or Action | Toning

DAY 21 is a FREE DAY

Your Secret to Feeling Great

Walking
30 Minutes, Monday through Saturday

Toning
Upper Body: 15–30 Minutes, Monday, Wednesday, and Friday
(using 1–10 pound hand weights)
Lower Body: 15–30 Minutes, Tuesday, Thursday, and Saturday
(using 1–2 pound ankle weights)
Sunday: Free day! Enjoy your favorite activity!

This is all you need to get started creating a new you!*

Upper Body Exercises
Monday, Wednesday, Friday, do 12 repetitions of each exercise, working your way up to 3 sets of 12 repetitions.

Exercise 1

Step 1

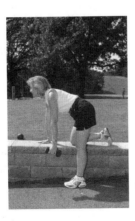

Starting position

Step 2

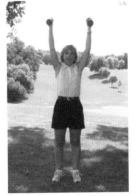

Reach hands straight up.

Exercise 2

Step 1

Starting position

Step 2

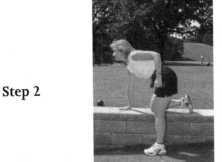

Bend elbow and draw back and up.
Complete set, then repeat using other arm.

*Consult your doctor before starting any exercise program.

Upper Body Exercises continued

Exercise 3

Step 1

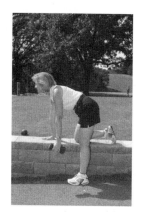

Starting position

Step 2

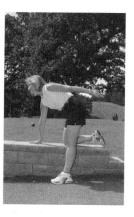

Draw straight arm back and up.
Complete set, then repeat using other arm.

Exercise 4

Step 1

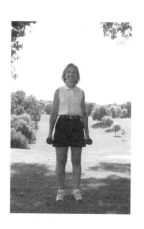

Starting position

Step 2

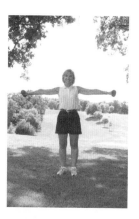

Lift arms up and out to shoulder height.

Exercise 5

Step 1

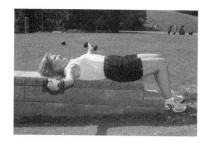

Starting position

Step 2

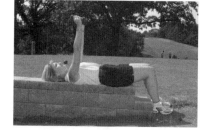

Bring straight arms upward and
bring hands together.

Exercise 6

Step 1

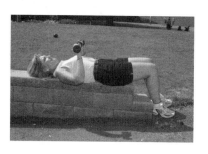

Starting position

Step 2

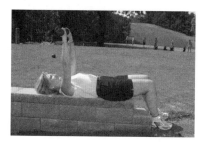

Push hands upward, straightening arms.

Upper Body Exercises continued

Exercise 7

Step 1

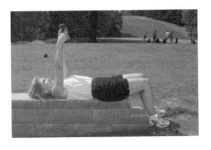

Starting position

Step 2

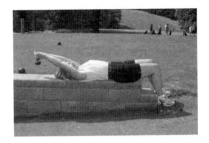

Draw straight arms back, above head.

Exercise 8

Step 1

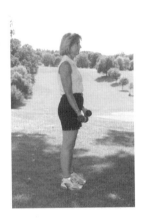

Starting position

Step 2

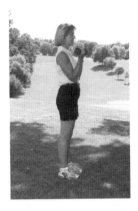

Bend elbows, raising weights to chest.

Lower Body Exercises

Tuesday, Thursday, Saturday, do 12 repetitions of each exercise, working your way up to 3 sets of 12 repetitions.

Exercise 1

Step 1

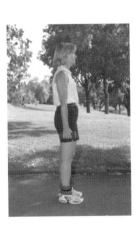

Starting position

Step 2

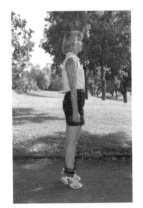

Lift heels off ground and hold briefly.

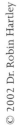

Lower Body Exercises continued

Exercise 2

Step 1
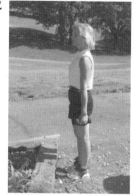
Starting position

Step 2
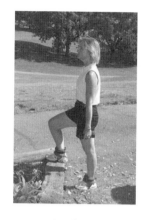
Raise right foot onto step

Step 3
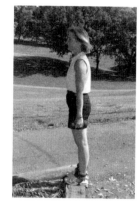
Raise left foot onto step. Return right foot, then left foot, to ground. Repeat steps, using left foot first.

Exercise 3

Step 1
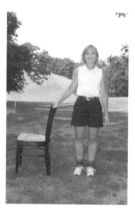
Starting position

Step 2
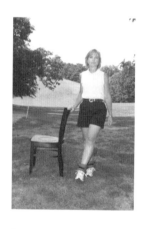
Raise foot and cross straight leg over balanced leg. Complete set, then repeat with other leg

Exercise 4

Step 1
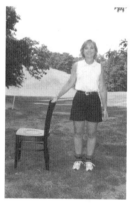
Starting position

Step 2
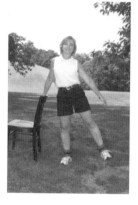
Raise straight arm and leg to side. Complete set, then repeat on other side

Lower Body Exercises continued

Exercise 5

Step 1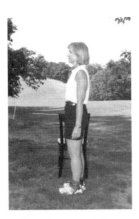

Step 2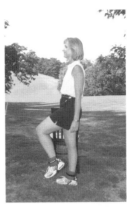

Starting position

Bend and lift knee. Complete set,
then repeat with opposite leg.

Exercise 6

Step 1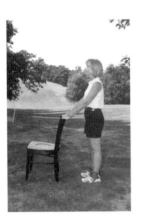

Step 2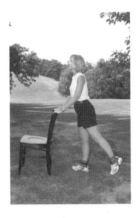

Starting position

Raise foot, keeping leg straight.
Complete set, then repeat with other leg.

Exercise 7

Step 1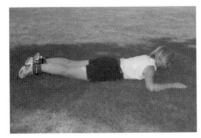

Step 2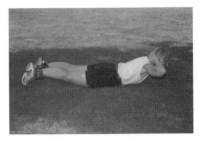

Starting position

Lift head and feet off of ground,
arching upward.

Exercise 8

Step 1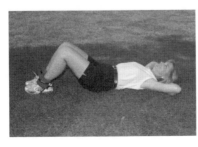

Step 2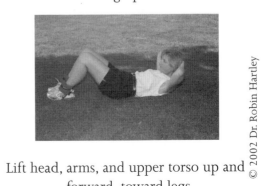

Starting position

Lift head, arms, and upper torso up and
forward, toward legs.